1971

THE REFERENCE SHELF   VOLUME 43 NUMBER 3

THE
NATION'S HEALTH

EDITED BY
STEPHEN LEWIN

THE H. W. WILSON COMPANY

NEW YORK   1971

THE REFERENCE SHELF

The books in this series contain reprints of articles, excerpts from books, and addresses on current issues and social trends in the United States and other countries. There are six separately bound numbers in each volume, all of which are generally published in the same calendar year. One number is a collection of recent speeches; each of the others is devoted to a single subject and gives background information and discussion from various points of view, concluding with a comprehensive bibliography. Books in the series may be purchased individually or on subscription.

THE NATION'S HEALTH

Copyright © 1971
By The H. W. Wilson Company

International Standard Book Number 0-8242-0448-4
Library of Congress Catalog Card Number 70-149385

PREFACE

For some time now it has been generally accepted by medical professionals that the health care system in the United States is in a state of chaos.

This may seem a strange statement, for the United States has long prided itself on the quality and ingenuity of its medical care. American doctors and researchers have pioneered in a multitude of medical breakthroughs, and our doctors routinely perform procedures today that would have been impossible or highly dangerous a few years ago. People come to our hospitals from all over the world for complex brain, heart, and other operations.

Yet, much of the day-to-day business of treating patients in the United States is inferior in quality, ridiculously expensive, and wasteful. Indeed, it has been said with some justification, that the United States is among the best places in the world to get really seriously ill, but one of the worst places to get just routinely sick.

It has been charged that the U.S. system of dispensing medical care is obsolete, overstrained, redundant, and exorbitant. Demand for care far outpaces the resources of the country to supply it. Although medical costs are soaring, hospital and medical schools throughout the country are on the verge of bankruptcy. Although there is a serious shortage of doctors in the United States, American medical schools are now turning away 60 per cent of the qualified applicants because of the lack of space. Despite the existence of costly government plans such as Medicare and Medicaid, and despite widespread public health insurance plans, many Americans could be financially destroyed by prolonged and serious illness in the family. For millions of Americans, going to the hospital means heavy, if not crushing expenses.

3

In some parts of the country, there is an oversupply of doctors. Yet many communities have been without a doctor for years. Inside almost any city, there is a grave imbalance in doctor supply. There may be block after block of offices of expensive specialists, yet a person living in that area may find it impossible to get a doctor to make a house visit.

It is not just the poor who suffer from inadequate medical care, although the poor too suffer. Middle-class people, and even the affluent, find it difficult to get a doctor for anything short of an emergency.

Why is it that there are inadequacies in a country that devotes such a vast proportion of its resources to the problem? This book is an attempt to deal with that question. The first section concerns the breakdown in the system of delivering medical care to the American people. The second discusses the changing role of the doctor. The third section examines the issue of national health insurance. The fourth deals with the relationship between medicine and the community. The fifth and final section discusses various sociomedical questions in the light of the changing values of American society.

The editor would like to thank the various authors, editors, and publishers who granted permission for use of material included in this book. He again is indebted to his wife, Deirdre, for her patience and help in the preparation of the book.

STEPHEN LEWIN

July 1971

CONTENTS

I. OUR SICK HEALTH CARE SYSTEM

EDITOR'S INTRODUCTION

If the solution to the ills of the U.S. medical care system was simply a matter of more money, these problems no doubt would have been solved long ago. But the problem is not just money. Perhaps it is not even mainly money, although more money will be needed to attack the problem. The United States already spends a total of $70 billion each year on health care. More than $21 billion of that sum comes from the Federal Government. The nation already devotes a larger share of its resources to health care—almost 7 per cent of its gross national product—than does any other industrialized country.

Yet the result is not equal to the outlay. By almost any statistical measure of health, the United States is being far outstripped in indices of health care by countries with far lower standards of living. We rank far behind many industrialized countries in terms of both male and female life expectancy, infant and maternal mortality, incidence of heart disease and other chronic ailments such as diabetes, and rejection of men by the armed forces for health reasons.

Some experts argue that these figures are less a reflection of the quality of care provided in the United States than of the personal life styles of Americans. Yet even some of the staunchest defenders of U.S. medicine are now arguing that something is seriously wrong with the provision of medical care to the American people. To many of them, something is needed other than the traditional "more money, more research, and more gadgets."

In the first selection in this section, President Richard M. Nixon outlines just how crucial is the problem of health care in the United States. In the President's view, the problem is of such a magnitude as to require not merely new programs and new money, but "a new approach which is equal to the complexity of the challenges." Next, Senator Abraham Ribicoff (Democrat) of Connecticut examines what he calls the myth of superior health care in the United States and reaches the conclusion that American medical care is distinctly inferior in almost every measurable way, with the exception of the price tag. The educational and financial problems of medical schools are the subject of the next selection, from the *National Observer*. The New York *Times* article on the report of the Carnegie Commission on Higher Education urges a turning away from the traditional emphasis on scientific research in the education of medical personnel to an approach centered on the delivery of health care in the most efficient manner. This is followed by a selection from a *Fortune* magazine article by John M. Mecklin that discusses the problems of hospitals today, pointing out why some hospitals are on the brink of disaster while others have never been in better financial health. The sixth selection, by medical writer Fred Anderson, staff associate of the National Academy of Engineering, examines the present system of providing care and suggests that the major evil lies in the present fee-for-service system under which the patient pays a fee for each office visit, home visit, X ray, or whatever service is provided. Anderson suggests that one answer may be in a system of medical prepayment. In the final selection, Elliot L. Richardson, Secretary of Health, Education, and Welfare, discusses the problems of health care as myth and reality.

TOWARDS A NEW HEALTH STRATEGY [1]

In the last twelve months alone, America's medical bill went up 11 per cent, from $63 [billion] to $70 billion. In the

[1] From President Nixon's message to Congress urging a new national health strategy in the United States, February 18, 1971. Text from New York *Times*. p 16. F. 19, '71.

last ten years, it has climbed 170 per cent, from the $26 billion level in 1960. Then we were spending 5.3 per cent of our gross national product on health; today we devote almost 7 per cent of our GNP to health expenditures.

This growing investment in health has been led by the Federal Government. In 1960, Washington spent $3.5 billion on medical needs—13 per cent of the total. This year it will spend $21 billion—or about 30 per cent of the nation's spending in this area.

But what are we getting for all this money?

For most Americans, the result of our expanded investment has been more medical care and care of higher quality. A profusion of impressive new techniques, powerful new drugs, and splendid new facilities has developed over the past decade. During that same time, there has been a 6 per cent drop in the number of days each year that Americans are disabled. Clearly there is much that is right with American medicine.

But there is also much that is wrong.

One of the biggest problems is that fully 60 per cent of the growth in medical expenditures in the last ten years has gone not for additional services but merely to meet price inflation. Since 1960, medical costs have gone up twice as fast as the cost of living. Hospital costs have risen five times as fast as other prices. For growing numbers of Americans, the cost of care is becoming prohibitive and even those who can afford most care may find themselves impoverished by a catastrophic medical expenditure.

The shortcomings of our health care system are manifested in other ways as well. For some Americans—especially those who live in remote rural areas or in the inner city—care is simply not available. The quality of medicine varies widely with geography and income. Primary-care physicians and outpatient facilities are in short supply in many areas and most of our people have trouble obtaining medical attention on short notice. Because we pay so little attention to preventing disease and treating it early, too many people get sick and need intensive treatment.

Things do not have to be this way. We can change these conditions—indeed, we must change them if we are to fulfill our promise as a nation. Good health care should be readily available to all of our citizens.

It will not be easy for our nation to achieve this goal. It will be impossible to achieve it without a new sense of purpose and a new spirit of discipline.

THE "HEALTHIEST NATION" MYTH [2]

About two years ago the wife of a forty-three-year-old house painter in Alabama was hospitalized for cancer of the cervix and colon while pregnant with the couple's fifth child. Over an eighteen-month period she had several major operations, round-the-clock nurses, and heavy dosages of expensive drugs, but she died. Her husband was left with a $30,000 medical bill, of which only $9,000 was covered by insurance.

Ruinous medical bills like this are only one example of what is wrong with American health care. (If the painter had lived in Sweden, which has national health insurance, his wife's hospital bill would have been $1.40 a day, doctors' visits would have cost $1.35 each, and drugs, if not free, would have been provided at minimal cost.) Another is that this woman was among 100,000 Americans who die of cancer each year who might be saved by earlier or better care.

There are serious and growing defects in American medicine. They range from shameful efforts at prevention—in which the patient is partly at fault—to a lack of manpower, equipment, and facilities, in which the patient clearly is a victim. From the patient's standpoint this translates to a fear that he will not find a doctor in an emergency, that he will receive inferior care, and that his rights as a consumer will be

[2] Article by Senator Abraham Ribicoff (Democrat, Connecticut). *Saturday Review*. 53:18-20. Ag. 22, '70. Copyright 1970 Saturday Review, Inc. Reprinted by permission.

ignored by physicians and other health professionals. (A Harris poll showed that 64 per cent of the public—nearly seven of every ten people—believed that "most doctors don't want you to bother them.")

These fears are well founded; many Americans, even when they can pay, cannot find a doctor. This shortage is due basically to the "professional birth control" the American Medical Association practiced in the 1930s and, more recently, to the development of specialists and the tendency of doctors to pursue careers in teaching, research, industry, and public health instead of patient care. Those who can't find a doctor generally descend on already overburdened hospital emergency rooms, with the result that only one third of the people waiting there for care are true emergency cases.

Those physicians we do have are distributed unevenly throughout the country and not necessarily according to need. A 1965 survey of 1,500 cities and towns in the upper Midwest showed that 1,000 had no doctor at all and 200 had only one. Highly populated areas have their problems as well. In Rochester, New York, the Monroe County Medical Society receives thirty to fifty calls every day from people looking for a doctor, according to Medical Society officials who testified during my 1968 Senate hearings on health care.

Yet, this year alone, medical schools turned down 15,000 well-qualified students who wanted places in freshman classes. There was only enough space for 10,000. That is an involuntary rejection rate of three of every five applicants, a loss this country cannot afford. And medical schools face such severe financial problems that 43 of 107 in the United States received "financial distress" grants from the Government. At the same time, cutbacks in Federal funds have limited construction money to one of every four potential new medical schools this year.

The best the Government's efforts for fiscal 1969 and 1970 will do is produce—by 1975 at the earliest—another 1,600 physicians, an increase of slightly more than one half of 1 per cent in the current physician population. In the meantime, as health coverage expands, the demand for more doctors will automatically increase. Unless the country is willing to provide significant incentives to correct the poor geographic distribution of physicians, the situation can only worsen for certain groups in the population. The picture would be even darker were it not for foreign medical graduates, who comprise 14 per cent of the nation's active physicians and 28 per cent of its interns and residents.

Specialized hospital expertise also is distributed unevenly. A 1967 report of the President's Commission on Heart Disease, Cancer, and Stroke surveyed the 777 U.S. hospitals equipped to perform open-heart surgery. Such operations are complicated and demanding, with constantly changing procedures that require frequent use and a well-trained staff. Nonetheless, a full one third of the hospitals surveyed by the commission had no open-heart surgery cases that year, more than 60 per cent had fewer than one a week, and 30 per cent had fewer than one a month.

Nor are hospital medical practice standards in general what they should be. The scandal of publicly owned hospitals has been well documented by young interns and residents, forcing the Joint Commission on the Accreditation of Hospitals to strip some large-city hospitals of their already minimal levels of accreditation and to threaten others with similar action. Also, physicians in voluntary, nonprofit hospitals admit privately that they cut too many corners and take too many chances with the lives and safety of patients.

There are stories of heart attack patients placed in halls near nurses' stations when cardiac units are full, of hospitals failing to separate infectious gynecological patients from obstetrics areas containing newborn infants, and special emergency units that function without any blood bank and that provide X-ray service only between 8 A.M. and 4 P.M. and not on weekends at all. It is impossible to ignore the warning from the chief of medicine at one of New York City's public hospitals: "You come to this hospital, and we're telling you somebody's going to take care of you. The fact is, you're going to lie in a pool of feces, develop an ulcer, septicemia [blood poisoning], and perhaps ultimately die because of inadequate nursing care."

The poor have known for years that medical care was expensive, hard to get, and uneven in quality. So has much of rural and small-town America. Now the urban middle class, which must receive its care from the same poorly organized system, is learning all this, too. Although high costs have hit harder than any other problem so far, the American middle class is beginning to understand that poor organization also can result in death or disability.

Obstetricians and pediatricians at one major teaching hospital insist that many infant deaths and cases of brain damage and blood disease could be prevented if communities devised better systems of identifying women who were "high-risk" pregnancies. What troubles these physicians is that such cases often are identifiable, the risk to the mother and child predictable, the treatment known, and the resources available.

Meanwhile, some individuals still contend that the medical crisis in this country is exaggerated and overblown, that the doctor shortage is not severe, and that many communities without doctors may be even healthier than those with doctors. But none of those individuals who argue this position is willing to live in a community without doctors. They point out that our finest medical care is second to none and that people from other countries come here for open-heart surgery as well as for complex brain and eye operations. But the shocking truth is that in too many instances it doesn't even extend beyond their own doorstep to the approximately twenty million Americans who receive inadequate care or no care at all.

Defenders of American medical care also argue that the Swedish system, good though it may seem, is not as cheap as it appears: The Swedish citizen pays 20 per cent of his taxes—

the highest in the world—for health. Even so, Sweden still devotes 1 per cent *less* of its gross national product and $45 *less* per person for health than does the United States.

If cost were any indication of quality, then America would be the healthiest nation in recorded history. We spend more money on health and medical care than any other people in the world: $63 billion a year, 6.7 per cent of our gross national product, $294 per person. No other country can match any of these figures.

But a dozen nations, each of which spends less per country and per person, can match us and do a better job of preventing infant deaths. Twelve nations also have a lower maternal mortality rate. In seventeen countries, men live longer than in the United States. Women have a better chance of surviving in ten other countries. And the percentage of men who will die between the ages of forty and fifty is less in seventeen other nations. Obviously, we are not the healthiest nation in the world. We are not even close. Personal habits, life-styles, education, income, genetics, and physical and social environment have combined, along with medical-care deficiencies, to produce the data that destroy this myth.

Medical care may play only a secondary role in these world rankings (although the countries that come out on top, such as Sweden, also have good and inexpensive medical care). Public health officials often contend they could do more for the nation's health by getting rid of the slums and ending pollution than by making sure everybody has a thorough physical exam once a year. Early death, they say, seems related more to income and life-style than to medical care. And although infant mortality occurs mostly among poor blacks, who often do not see a doctor, a recent California study found that whites with regular medical care do not have that state's lowest infant death rate. Japanese-Americans do. In fact, they outrank whites on every index of good health.

But none of these considerations should obscure or minimize the point that when most Americans speak of health they mean medical care, because that is what the $63 billion is supposed to buy. Nor can we minimize the fact that health costs continue to rise out of proportion to other prices, and that few signs of relief are visible on the manpower horizon. Just five years ago the national health bill was a fraction of today's $63 billion figure—$37 billion. Rough estimates predict that it will reach $100 billion in the next five years and may even double and reach $200 billion in the early 1980s.

If current trends continue, the major share of that increase—47 per cent in the past—will be due to rising prices caused by inflation, technology, long-overdue wage increases for hospital employees from nurses to kitchen workers, and just plain higher charges. Thirty-five per cent will come from more services provided per person, and 18 per cent from population increases. Hospital charges, which doubled between 1956 and 1966, already have gone up another 50 per cent in the last three years. Doctors' fees during the 1960s rose twice as fast as the general cost of living, with the biggest boost coming since the advent of Medicare.

A reliable prediction—one that a health economist would stand by—is not available. Too many political uncertainties cloud the picture. But no special wisdom is needed to understand that unless efficiencies and controls are adopted, the cost of health care will skyrocket out of sight. Reliable predictions of medical manpower needs also depend upon basic decisions the country makes regarding the organization, financing, and delivery of medical care. But all the evidence suggests that manpower shortages will continue.

This, then, is where we stand today: high costs, not enough doctors, nurses, or other health professionals, too many people receiving poor care or no care at all, inadequate health insurance, and most medical care organized and operated in a manner that rewards inefficiencies and perpetuates inequities. All that keeps the medical care system afloat, as Dr. John Knowles [general director, Massachusetts General Hospital] suggested at my 1968 hearings, is the fact that millions literally have no knowledge of their medical needs.

Thus, when one large metropolitan hospital recently gave medical examinations in a ghetto junior high school, 20 per cent of the students were found to have hearing and sight problems. Because nobody had ever examined them before, many had spent half their public school lives in schools for the retarded.

The same type of problem shows up again when eye examinations are given suburban children. The National Center for Health Statistics estimated that in 1967 nearly half the people in this country had at least one chronic disease or impairment.

Why should these conditions exist? Why should medical care be on the verge of collapse for so many Americans?

One compelling reason was contained in a letter last fall from the Department of Health, Education, and Welfare. I had asked how each of the twenty-four departments and agencies that spend the Government's $20.6 billion health budget contributed to the formulation and implementation of the national health policy. With refreshing candor, HEW answered: "Up to and including the present there has never been a formulation of national health policy as such. In addition, no specific mechanism has been set up to carry out this function."

That in itself is an intolerable situation. If there is no policy, there can be no goals. If there are no goals, there can be no strategies. This is what we have today, and the result is that medical care, instead of being a public responsibility, is a private business. It is operated more for the convenience of its practitioners than according to the needs of the sick.

Washington's $20.6 billion health budget is one third the money the United States spends on health. Clearly, the Government has both the potential and the responsibility to spend its money as a lever for improvements in manpower, organization, and efficiency in addition to whatever action is taken on national health insurance.

If Washington does not assure all Americans access to adequate medical care at a cost they can afford, with enough manpower to meet their needs, then who will? If Washington does not act, then the best advice anyone can offer is this: Get sick today; don't wait five years.

GRIM DIAGNOSIS FOR MEDICAL SCHOOLS [3]

The nation's medical schools are sick and getting sicker. Unable to cure their ills, some are close to giving up the ghost. It is hard to exaggerate the distress—or minimize the effects the crisis could have on American medicine.

The immediate, most obvious problem is money. Medical schools have been badly lacerated by sharp cutbacks in Federal funds at the same time that their costs have been zooming. Sixty-one of the country's 107 medical schools (with 379 affiliated teaching hospitals) have received or are receiving Federal "distress" funds to help meet operating deficits.

A quick money transfusion would help; in fact, it may be the difference between life and death for some schools. But the root causes of the distress go deeper. The schools are finding it increasingly difficult to keep up with demands being made upon them: more doctors, more and better health care, maintaining research on medical frontiers, and more effective methods of administering resources.

Ironically, one reason for the upsurge in costs is that medical schools have been increasing enrollments in response to Government pleas for help in solving the nation's doctor shortage. It's figured the country needs 50,000 more physicians than it has today.

[3] From "Sick Medical Schools Receive Emergency Help," by Jim Hampton, news editor. *National Observer.* p 1+. N. 16, '70. Reprinted by permission.

Among the schools hardest hit are:

Case Western Reserve University, Cleveland, which dipped into endowment funds for $12 million before being rescued—temporarily at least—by a $3 million grant this year from the Ohio legislature

St. Louis University, which is keeping its medical school afloat with funds freed up by closing its dental, aviation technology, and engineering schools. The 140-year-old school is so pinched, says Dean Robert H. Felix, that it may not be able to admit a first-year class in 1971.

New York Medical College, which required a $500,000 Federal distress loan to break even this year even though it mortgaged property for $10 million and is spending $6 million in endowment money

Georgetown University and George Washington University, both in Washington, D.C., say their schools may close unless Congress, which is the District of Columbia's "legislature," antes up money to cover Georgetown's projected $1.42 million deficit and George Washington's $1,991,159 anticipated deficit.

Marquette University's medical school became the Medical College of Wisconsin after it was rescued from bankruptcy by a $3.2 million emergency grant from the Wisconsin legislature.

Financial anemia, respecter neither of age nor of reputation, threatens the Johns Hopkins University School of Medicine, for seventy years one of the world's premier medical schools. The school ran $910,000 into the red last year. This year its deficit will more than double, to an anticipated $2.234 million.

This rate of deficit spending would bankrupt the medical school if left unstemmed. "If you take the most conservative view, we could only continue a few years at the present rate," says Dr. Lincoln Gordon, the university's president. Adds

Dr. David E. Rogers, medical-school dean at Johns Hopkins: "It may take the closing of several medical schools to get the [Nixon] Administration to take notice."

In 1958-59 the Federal Government gave medical schools about $95 million, approximately 30 per cent of their budgets, in grants for research, training of specialists, teaching, and the like. A decade later the Federal contribution was around $700 million. Research grants had increased 426 per cent, training and other grants had zoomed 613 per cent.

The Federal share of all medical schools' budgets thus rose to 53 per cent. At some schools—notably the better ones, like Hopkins, with big-name faculty—it was somewhat higher. Moreover, at some schools—Hopkins included—the Federal Government was putting up $4 of every $5 spent for medical research.

Things began souring in the twilight of the Johnson Administration. Pressed by inflation, costs of the Vietnam war, unanticipated spending on Medicare and Medicaid, and a general decline in enthusiasm for scientific endeavors, the Government dropped medicine's priority several notches.

"Special Grants" Keep Doors Open

Last year [1969] HEW gave 72 medical schools 95 "special projects" grants totaling $34.7 million. These grants were conceived primarily for curriculum improvements, but 61 of the schools applied them to operating costs. Among them were 32 schools deemed in "serious financial need." This year HEW spread a total of $15 million—about the same given the 32 schools last year—among 43 schools in similar straits. . . .

At Johns Hopkins in Baltimore, the effects of Federal cutbacks show up dramatically. Hopkins' experiences probably also illustrate, as well as any one school can, what the reliance on Federal money has wrought.

"We're Pretty Vulnerable"

Hopkins is spending $34 million this year. Of this, $22 million—or 60 per cent—comes from NIH [National Institutes of Health, HEW agency established April 1968] mostly for research. "We're pretty vulnerable," says Dean Rogers. "The better the medical school, the higher the percentage of Federal funding."

Last year [1969] Johns Hopkins lost $1.6 million in Federal money, including $600,000 for projects that were approved by NIH but never financed. The other $1 million was lost through "negotiated reductions."

In happier days, NIH approved Hopkins' grant applications 70 to 75 per cent of the time, says Dr. Rogers. No more: The rate is now 40 to 50 per cent. This has two disturbing effects. First, it makes grants harder to get by young, unknown doctors. Second, it jeopardizes projects to which Hopkins has committed itself for years on the basis of previous NIH support.

"It takes fifteen to twenty years to build up a top-flight biomedical team," Dr. Rogers stresses, "but you can tear one down in six months." That's in danger of happening here now. One professor has been working since 1950 on research involving metabolism, heart disease, and diabetes.

But now his NIH grant has been cut off. Several assistants have had to be dropped and, when the school's emergency funds run out shortly, his work will come to an end.

Future Leadership Crimped

Training programs also are hurting. . . . [In 1969] Hopkins lost $375,061 in Federal training grants. This money would have supported postresidency training in cardiology, physiology, and pharmacology. "This has been our underpinning for training the new leadership of medicine, the future teachers and future researchers," Dr. Rogers says.

Medical schools generally are making tremendous efforts to admit more students from working-class backgrounds and minority groups. . . . [In 1969] Hopkins had 391 students, of whom 55 per cent had to have loans or grants to meet expenses. This year's [1970] class is up to 420, and 45 per cent of its students come from families with incomes of less than $12,000 a year. . . .

Making medical education accessible to poor people and minorities is a social imperative, authorities agree. But it also exacerbates the medical school's financial problems. "It usually costs about twice as much to keep these students in school because their financial background is not as good," says Dr. Cooper. "With inadequate loan and scholarship funds," because of Federal cutbacks in those categories, "the schools have been digging into whatever reserves and endowment funds they have."

"A Crunch" for Scholars

Here at Hopkins, the loan-scholarship situation is creating a "terrific crunch," Dean Rogers says. Tuition is $2,000 a year now and will rise to $2,500 next fall, but tuition pays only a fraction of a medical student's education. . . .

[Hopkins officials emphasize] that the only long-range solution is more Federal aid to all medical schools.

"Medical schools are a precious national resource," says Dr. Rogers, "and to pretend that they could float along on money available from the private sector is silly. It just couldn't be done."

Some medical educators think it was a mistake for the schools to become so dependent on Federal money. Not Dr. Rogers. "Without Federal money, a lot of private medical schools would have withered on the vine; they would have closed."

Many medical schools, like Hopkins, are preparing for lean years. Dr. Rogers has let six faculty members go and will not fill twelve other posts when they become vacant.

"Deficits don't only show up in dollars, you know, says pipe-smoking Dr. Gordon. To which Dr. Russell Ne son, president of John Hopkins Hospital, adds:

"There is an enormous bill that has to be paid her sometime, by some generation."

REVAMPING OUR MEDICAL SCHOOLS [4]

The United States today faces only one serious man power shortage, and that is in health care personnel. Th shortage can become even more acute as health insuranc expands, leading to even more unmet needs and greate cost inflation, unless corrective action is taken now. It take a long lead time to get more doctors and dentists.

Higher education, as it trains the most skilled healt personnel, has a great responsibility for the welfare of th nation. What colleges of agriculture once did for a rura society can now be done for an urban society by the healt science centers—and that is to improve the quality of lif for nearly all people in their areas.

Flexner Model's Flaws

The Flexner model [of medical education in the Unite States] (suggested by Dr. Abraham Flexner sixty years ago based on Johns Hopkins, Harvard, and, before them, Ge man medical education, called for emphasis on biologica research. Science was to be at the base of medical educa tion. The Flexner model has been the sole fully accepte model in the United States since 1910. Some schools hav fulfilled its promise brilliantly; others have been pale imita tions; but all have tried to follow it. It has led to grea strides forward in the quality of research and the qualit of individual medical practitioners.

The Flexner, or *research* model, however, looked in ward to science in the medical school itself. It is a sel

[4] From "Excerpts from the Carnegie Commission's Report on Medical Edu cation in U.S." New York *Times.* p 16. O. 30, '70. © 1970 by The New Yor Times Company. Reprinted by permission.

ontained approach. Consequently, it has two weaknesses
n modern times: (1) it largely ignores health care delivery
utside the medical school and its own hospital; and (2)
t sets science in the medical school apart from science on
he general campus with resulting duplication of effort.

This second weakness is now being highlighted by the
extension of medical concern beyond science into economics,
ociology, engineering, and many other fields. Medical
chools have had their own departments of biochemistry,
but to add their own departments of economics and sociology
and engineering would accentuate the problem of duplica-
ion of faculty and equipment.

Also, the better economists would rather be in a department of economics on a general campus than separated
rom their colleagues in a department of medical economics:
members of other disciplines would have similar prefer-
ences. The self-contained Flexner model thus leads to expensive duplication and can lead to some loss in quality.

Two new models are arising: (1) the *health care delivery*
model, where the medical school, in addition to training,
does research in health care delivery, advises local hospitals
and health authorities, works with community colleges and
comprehensive colleges on the training of allied health personnel, carries on continuing education for health personnel, and generally orients itself to external service; and
(2) the *integrated science* model, where most or all of the
basic science (and social science) instruction is carried on
within the main campus (or other general campuses) and
not duplicated in the medical school, which provides mainly
clinical instruction. In this model (as in England), the
medical school may be, essentially, a teaching hospital; but
this is not necessary—it may, rather, carry on all its "Flexner" functions except the traditional first one or two years
of science education.

Different Directions

A few schools, and many parts of schools, will, and should, stay with the Flexner model, but we believe tha the nation will be better served as many schools move in different directions. A diversity of models and mixture of models is now desirable.

Not only can the developing and new schools experiment; but as exciting schools expand, they can direct their expansion in new directions so that there can be diversity *within* schools—for example, the next group of forty additional students admitted might be asked to take their science on the main campus of the parent university. The "cluster-college" approach of changing and diversifying—rather than just duplicating on a larger scale—when expanding a general campus can be undertaken also in a health science center.

OUR SICK HOSPITALS [5]

Not long ago, when Americans who were not charity cases entered a hospital, they faced the prospect of serious financial loss, or even financial catastrophe. Now the advent of private insurance plans and of Government assistance through Medicare and Medicaid has changed all that. The doors of hospitals have swung open virtually to everyone. Only in relatively rare cases, where hospital stays are exceptionally prolonged, need a patient fear disastrous financial consequences.

But that indisputably progressive development has brought with it a new set of dangers. The hospital system itself is straining under the weight of the new loads imposed upon it. A new kind of financial catastrophe threatens—evidenced most graphically in the national average cost-per-patient day in general hospitals, which jumped

[5] From "Hospitals Need Management Even More Than Money" by John M. Mecklin, member of *Fortune* Board of Editors. *Fortune*. 81:96-9+. Ja. '70. Courtesy of Fortune Magazine.

rom $48.15 in 1966 to an estimated $67.60 in 1969. Pro-
ections indicate that the cost will reach about $74 this
ear. In some of our great medical centers the cost of a
patient day can run as high as $166, and that doesn't in-
lude the doctors' fees.

Such increases reflect the pressure of increased de-
nand, stimulated by insurance coverage, on relatively
tatic supply. The trend toward shorter hospital stays
hat accompanied improvements in the quality of medical
are has now been reversed. The average stay in a hosital is 8.4 days, almost a full day longer than it was
ight years ago. Big pushes on costs have come from the
ncreased wages of notoriously underpaid hospital em-
loyees: in three years, labor costs have climbed sharply,
specially in a few unionized areas such as New York
ity, where they have gone up more than 40 per cent.
alaries of interns and residents have shot up, as can be
een by the experience of one of the nation's leading hositals, Boston's Massachusetts General. At the same time,
ew technology requires the investment of more and more
apital. In sum, this hemorrhage of rising costs has sent
nsurance premiums soaring, and has presented legislators
nd taxpayers with the prospect of larger and larger out-
ays for government-sponsored programs. Medicare and
Medicaid alone are expected to pay hospitals more than
6 billion in 1970.

The inflation of some hospital costs might have been
etter contained by better management. But the man-
gers of many hospitals were ill-prepared for the explo-
ive new demand. Accounting methods have remained
nadequate. Construction of hospitals over the years has
een haphazard, so that costly facilities are often dupli-
ated by neighboring institutions. Yet the system also faces
n urgent need for some $7 billion in new capital to
modernize existing plant, plus about $3 billion more for
ome 90,000 additional beds in poorly served communities.

Hospitals cannot raise anywhere near these amounts b their own efforts.

In the search for more efficient and productive use c existing facilities, some hospitals are generating imagina tive new managerial approaches. They are using scientifi planning methods, and extending their use of computer into many new areas. A few institutions, such as Baptis Memorial Hospital in Memphis, have gone into sidelin business ventures to boost their incomes, and thus reduc the fees they must charge their patients.

But basic structural reforms are needed to give th system permanent stability. The immediate requiremen is certainly to revise the nature of insurance coverag(rewriting insurance plans so that they reward hospita economies and penalize waste. This, in turn, must be ac companied by widespread acceleration of a trend alread started—toward construction of separate, hospital-cor nected clinics, and other facilities for less intensive, an therefore less expensive, care. Clinics to provide ambu latory care, both in rural areas and in the core citie: could vastly relieve the pressure on hospitals. Sucl changes will become more urgent over the next few year: as a new wave of demand for care, mostly from the poo breaks over the present means for distributing it. . . .

From "Pesthouses" to Citadels of Science

The weaknesses of management and organization no coming to light in many of the nation's 7,137 hospita have their origins back in the nineteenth century. In thos days, hospitals were supported by charity and were com monly known as "pesthouses," places to dump the indigen sick while the rich were cared for in their own home where there was less danger of infection. As time changed, hospitals were transformed into citadels of mod ern science. But the old economic structure remained Today 34 per cent of the nation's hospital beds are in "vol

ntary," tax-free institutions that handle both paying and
harity cases; 11.5 per cent are in state-, county-, or munici-
al-owned establishments; and 2.9 per cent are in privately
wned hospitals operated for profit. The balance of 51.6
er cent of the beds are in various specialized institutions
uch as veterans' hospitals and facilities for psychiatric
nd tubercular care. The voluntary hospitals have emerged
s the most important segment of the industry. They are
he most advanced kinds of hospitals in medical skill, but
heir economics often are makeshift.

Initially, the voluntary hospitals relied almost entirely
n private gifts for capital needs. More recently, the main
ources have been government grants, and an allowance
or depreciation and interest costs in insurance payments.
But this has not been sufficient to meet the requirements
f a swiftly changing industry, and many hospitals have
een forced to hobble along with antiquated plant and
quipment, which adds substantially to their costs. Being
rivate institutions, voluntary hospitals are not required
o account to the general public, and some of them still
eep their books secret. Accounting methods often are an
stonishing jumble (in some cases nurses do the paper
ork in their spare time), although they have been im-
roved by the standardized requirements of Medicare and
Medicaid. . . .

On a more positive note, individual hospitals all over
he country have been coming up with ingenious programs
or making the existing system work better. . . . One approach, pioneered by Henry Ford Hospital—a 1,050-bed
oluntary institution with a large outpatient clinic in
Detroit—has been adopted by about a dozen hospitals elsewhere. It departs from the usual practice, where doctors
ther than the top administrators are associated with the
ospital, but work on the basis of the fees they charge
atients. Instead, all the doctors at Ford are full-time staff

members, working on salary. The hospital collects all fee
The system creates an incentive to be efficient, since the sta
has a stake in the success of the hospital's overall perform
ance. Unlike most voluntary hospitals, Ford has been able t
do without charitable contributions since 1950. . . .

Instant History

Computers, of course, have long been used in hospita
accounting. Now they are being introduced more directl
to serve the cause of patient care. One such system, de
veloped by National Data Communications, is being teste
at Baptist Hospital in Beaumont, Texas. Complete data o
each patient is fed into a computer through a push-butto
console when he is admitted to the hospital. The physicia
or nurse thereafter registers all new information, such a
prescribed treatments, so that everything about the patien
can be obtained quickly by asking the computer for a di
play or printout. The system also automatically perform
such chores as printing the gummed label to go with med
cation as soon as the order is received, and telling the stoc
room when the supply of an item should be replenished. I
can also be programmed to alert the nurse fifteen minute
before medication should be administered. . . .

Designed for Therapy

Better planning and better design of hospitals also prom
ise new efficiencies. New York Hospital recently conducted
study showing that better architectural planning could cut
nurse's daily walking distance by as much as 50 per cen
Hospitals generally are switching to single-room accom
modations, partly because of patient demands for greate
privacy, but also because of the discovery that being in
single room helps a patient get well faster. Memphis' Bap
tist Hospital has determined that a patient who needs eigh
days in a ward usually gets well in about seven days in
single room. . . .

Care for the Poor

Studies show that today the poor usually put health at least fourth in their priorities, after a job, education for the children, and housing. One of the nation's most aggressive leaders in the battle for better care for the poor has been Dr. John Knowles of Massachusetts General Hospital. Knowles estimated in 1968 that some 40,000 people in the Greater Boston area were suffering from untreated tuberculosis.

In various public statements, Knowles has repeatedly exhorted the medical world to serve the needs of the community as a whole, instead of catering only to patients who come to the hospital door. He estimates that hospital admissions from inner-city, impoverished communities could be cut as much as 80 per cent by preventing disease before it happens. The need, says Knowles, is "the development of comprehensive services, hospital based, extending all the expertise and the resources of the hospital out into community health centers in conjunction with local care institutions and stimulated through Federal legislation."

Something of the kind of operation that men like Knowles are looking for can be found in the huge system of 166 hospitals and 650,000 patients run by the Veterans Administration at an annual cost of $1.6 billion. Since they are primarily concerned with the care of veterans, VA hospitals are far from typical, with average patient stays of three to four weeks. But the system itself is widely admired among civilian hospital administrators. Through bulk procurement of supplies and advanced, heavily computerized management techniques,it keeps its costs to an impressive national average of about $40 per patient a day. But its main contribution to hospital doctrine has been the "whole man" concept—the idea that each eligible veteran not only should be treated when he comes to the hospital, but that it is the system's responsibility to try to prevent him from getting sick in the first place. To achieve this, the VA gives a total examination to every man admitted, to look for troubles of which he may not be aware. It tries to get veterans to come in regularly for checkups through repeated reminders of their right to free care.

In a number of other countries the medical system, including the hospitals, provides this kind of total care. The United States has the economic wealth to do just as well.

PAYING MORE, GETTING LESS [6]

[In 1969] President Nixon, [former] Secretary [of Health, Education, and Welfare Robert] Finch and the Assistant Secretary for Health and Scientific Affairs, Dr. Roger Egeberg, gathered at the White House to tell the nation that it is about to face a complete breakdown in the delivery of health services. Many think the breakdown has already occurred. Long waits for an appointment with a physician, poor service, and astronomical medical bills have gradually become the rule, rather than the exception. The public does not understand how this state of affairs came about, nor why physicians, hospitals and insurers have not done something about it. Particularly irritating is the Federal Government's failure, though it paid 29.6 per cent of the $53.1 billion spent on health in 1968. Long hours in the "waiting room," hurried and impersonal attention, difficulty in obtaining night and weekend care, reduction of services because staff is not available, high drug and treatment costs, loopholes in insurance coverage, and the like, tell only part of the story. The rest is told by statistics which smash any remaining confidence that we lead the world in health care. Fifteen other countries have longer average life expectancies. (Ten-year-old females have a longer life expectancy in twelve other countries, while the American male child of ten years is bested in thirty-one countries.) Infant mortality is less in fourteen other nations. Five

[6] From Part I of "The Growing Pains of Medical Care," a three-part article by Fred Anderson, staff associate of the National Academy of Engineering. *New Republic*. 162:15-17. Ja. 17, '70. Reprinted by Permission of The New Republic, © 1970, Harrison-Blaine of New Jersey, Inc.

countries have better maternal mortality rates. Twelve have better records for ulcers, diabetes, cirrhosis of the liver, hypertension without heart involvement. Twenty have less heart disease.

Whatever life expectancy a white American has, subtract seven years from the life of his nonwhite counterpart. Infant mortality rates are two times as great for nonwhites as for whites. Infant mortality rates for Negro children in Mississippi or a northern city are comparable to Ecuador's; nationwide, to Costa Rica's. Nonwhite maternal mortality is four times as great as the white rate. (The disparity in maternal death rates has grown from twofold to fourfold since the end of World War II.) In the city slums there is three times as much heart disease, five times as much mental disease, four times as much high blood pressure, and four times as many deaths before age thirty-five than there is nationwide.

The National Advisory Commission on Health Manpower (1967) reviewed fifteen representative studies of the quality of health care services in the United States. Here are the findings in three of the studies: (1) a survey of medical laboratories sponsored by the National Center for Communicable Diseases (United States Public Health Service) found that 25 per cent of reported laboratory results on known samples were erroneous; (2) an evaluation of all major female pelvic surgery performed during a six-month period in a community hospital revealed that 70 per cent of the operations which resulted in castration or sterilization were unjustified in the opinion of expert consultants; (3) the medical records of a random sample of 430 patients admitted to ninety-eight different hospitals in New York City during May 1962 were reviewed by expert clinicians. In their opinion only 57 per cent of all patients, and only 31 per cent of the general medical cases, received "optimal" care.

Organized medicine attributes deterioration in health care to our failure to produce enough physicians for the

growing demands for services. That's correct, to a point.
Over the decade 1955-1965 "physician-directed services"
rose 81 per cent and hospital services 65 per cent, although
the increased output of physicians (22 per cent) barely
exceeded population growth (17 per cent). In fact, the
increase in physicians who went into patient care (12 per
cent) was *less* than population growth. Thus the availability
of direct, personal treatment by a physician has diminished
at a time when demand for medical care is going up rapidly.
Demand has been so great that the expected undersupply
of physicians should have occurred years ago. What happened? Physicians learned to delegate many tasks to other
medical professionals, a practice which should be encouraged. Between 1955 and 1965, professional nurses increased
by 44 per cent, nonprofessional nurses 63 per cent, X-ray
technologists 56 per cent, and clinical laboratory personnel
70 per cent. Nevertheless, in the opinion of the National
Advisory Commission on Health Manpower, the existing
organization of medical care will soon require more physicians than the medical schools are capable of producing.
"If additional personnel are employed in the present manner and within present patterns and 'systems' of care," said
the Commission, "they will not avert, or even perhaps
alleviate, the crisis." That seems to say that no number
of additional physicians will be sufficient unless medical
care is reorganized. But the Commission did not say how
reorganization should be carried out.

What is so unsatisfactory about the organization of
our present medical care system? It consists by and large
of physicians in practice alone, or in small groups, on a
fee-for-service basis. The model is the independent business
entrepreneur, and a strong sense of nineteenth century in-
dividualism still guides professional conduct. (About 60
per cent of physicians in direct care of patients are solo
practitioners, even though less than 2 per cent of current
graduates go into general practice. Of physicians in office
practice, about 72 per cent still work on a fee-for-service

basis.) The "nonsystem" of separate practitioners and few
hospitals which grew up in the last century has somehow
managed to underpin the vast array of interlocking referrals, specialities, clinics, hospital services and financial ar-
rangements which exists today. That foundation is crum-
bling.

We cannot allow the further duplication of services,
equipment and personnel, not only because of the high
cost of redundancy, but because fee-for-service medicine
is medically one-sided. It is adequate for episodic care for
patients with a specific complaint. But such care, though
good, is delivered in sporadic bursts. It is not the per-
sonalized, lifelong program of prevention, diagnosis, treatment and rehabilitation that it should be. Patients very
rarely receive preventive screening or treatment. How could
a fee-for-service bill be written for "diagnosing" and pub-
licizing a dangerous playground? Who would be billed? The
city? Parents? Fixing up several broken arms is a medical
"service," with a going rate per arm. Getting embroiled with
nonmedical "playground" issues is not, even though the
expense of an ounce of prevention may be less than that
for a pound of cure.

It is not quite fair to lay all the ills of the health care
system at the feet of the practitioners who favor the fee-
for-service system. The American Medical Association, as
chief defender of fee-for-service, is almost a caricature of an
Establishment, an easy target. But medicine has two Establishments, both of which contribute to our troubles. The
second Establishment, hostile to the first, is based in urban
hospitals. It is research and technology oriented, often
salaried, and provides the world's best surgery and treatment for complex illnesses. The result is that though this
is the best country in the world in which to have a serious
illness, it is one of the worst countries in the world in
which to have a nonserious illness. That part of medicine
which most people encounter most often is mediocre. At
the same time, we have outstanding open-heart surgery, plas-

tic surgery, surgical organ transplantation, and diagnostic skills. It is this paradox which makes it possible for a patient to read in the waiting room literature of America's latest triumph of medical technology, while failing to receive quick, effective and inexpensive treatment for a sore throat.

The strength of the new hospital-based Establishment is in its domination of the medical schools. Dr. Charles E. Lewis of Harvard's Center for Community Medicine and Medical Care believes that the inertia of medical schools and their affiliated teaching hospitals is the health care delivery system's chief problem. The schools and their hospitals turn out excellent clinicians, scientifically imaginative researchers, who appear more concerned with a patient's interesting electrolytes than with his humdrum good health. A department chairman, selected perhaps, because he discovered subtle mechanisms of kidney function, makes the school's reputation (and much of its money) by his work and by the grants which he gets for research. No one can tell the collection of department chairmen who run a medical school, or their granting agencies, that the funds which they collect should go to teach students how to care for whole patients in the environment in which patients live.

MYTH AND REALITY IN HEALTH CARE [7]

Social issues are often shrouded in myth and misconception. As an example, for too long it was popularly believed that fathers of welfare families irresponsibly abandoned their wives and children to live carefree, devil-may-care lives financed by the public's largesse. But careful analyses by social scientists revealed that, in fact, able-bodied men on welfare were often forced by the system to leave their families.

[7] From "Myth and Reality: Problems of Health Care" by Elliot L. Richardson, Secretary of Health, Education, and Welfare. New York *Times*. p 39. Ap. 2, '71. Copyright © 1971 by The New York Times Company. Reprinted by permission.

Health care in the United States is a current example of a vast social issue encrusted with a layer of invention and illusion. We all know there is something wrong with the current health care system, and it is commonly held that too few doctors, greedy insurance companies, and an apathetic Government are at fault. But are these the real problems? Does such conventional "wisdom" mislead us to propose inadequate solutions to complex problems? Let us examine some of the nation's health myths in order to see the Administration's health proposals in light of the true problems behind them.

Myth: The United States is the only major industrial nation in the world that does not have a national health service or a program of nationalized health insurance. This claim was made last month on the floor of Congress, and the idea is widely shared, even among some health "experts." Those who hold this view seem to have in mind the British and Eastern European model in which health services are paid for out of general tax revenues. But the British model is not the typical Western European model. In fact, continental health insurance schemes are predominantly financed by employer-employee contributions and operate within the framework of national standards. This is basically the route the President has proposed that we travel—national health insurance, not nationalized health insurance.

Myth: There is a gross shortage of doctors in America. In fact, we have one of the highest ratios of doctors per capita in the world—and the number of physicians is growing at a rate faster than the population. The basic problem is maldistribution. There are too few doctors in the ghettos, in rural America and in the primary care disciplines, such as general practice and pediatrics, while there is no real shortage of doctors in suburban practices or in certain specialties like surgery. To meet this paradox of scarcity amid plenitude, the Administration has proposed incentives to bring doctors to the areas and types of practice where they are most needed.

Myth: It is better doctoring that is making us a healthier nation. In fact, infant mortality rates have declined and longevity has increased due largely to better nutrition and sanitation, higher income, and improved education. For example, when we replaced the horse and buggy, the death rate of infants and children fell because of an accompanying decline in fatal diarrhea caused by animal filth. In recognition of these interrelationships, the Administration has proposed efforts to clean our environment, provide a basic income for poor families, provide adequate nutrition, and make education available to more people. In truth, the Administration is concerned about health and not only medical care. That is one reason why we feel that very expensive federally financed health insurance schemes may, in fact, preempt too large a share of Federal tax revenues for medical care, when a more balanced approach would better achieve health goals.

Myth: Insurance companies are getting fat on health insurance. In reality, these companies on the average have retained less than 6 per cent of premiums for administrative overhead and profit on group health insurance. The Administration's choice to build upon the present strengths of our system was based on a desire to reform, not dismantle, our health care institutions. We see no need to create another mammoth bureaucracy in response to the misconception that we are making the rich richer.

An Old Saying: "An ounce of prevention is worth a pound of cure." Not all ancient wisdom is a myth. Prevention is a more satisfactory solution than cure. It can be demonstrated that significant improvements in our health status will come about more through prevention of accidents and chronic disease than through improvements in curative medicine. The President's proposed health education, accident prevention, and biomedical research programs are targeted at those areas of prevention where we can hope to have the greatest success.

With our health program we have attempted to eschew the simple, grant solution, which often turns out to be both expensive and misdirected. A hallmark of a responsible government is the ability to distinguish between sound reasoning and chimeras.

II. THE DOCTOR AND HIS PRACTICE

EDITOR'S INTRODUCTION

The doctor is the central figure in medicine. He and he alone determines what treatment is given a patient and how long it lasts. He determines the drugs used and the experts consulted, and, in the absence of consumer groups or governmental control, he is almost unchallenged in determining the cost.

The most obvious fact about doctors today in the United States is that there aren't enough of them. There are about 300,000 doctors in the country; by itself, this is an acceptable if not entirely satisfactory figure. However, only about two thirds of them actually treat patients. The remainder are either retired or they are in medical administration, teaching, or research.

Even then, the doctors who are in practice are unevenly distributed in terms of the people to be treated. Some areas of a city are well provided with doctors' offices, but a slum in that city may have a doctor-patient ratio of one to 20,000 or 30,000. The same disproportion works against people in rural areas where the nearest doctor may be too remote to be much use in an emergency.

This section examines the often difficult, often lucrative, role of the doctor in the U.S. system of medical care. In the first selection, Dr. John H. Knowles, general director of the Massachusetts General Hospital in Boston, takes doctors to task for failing "to meet the public demand for cost controls and comprehensive health insurance, high and uniform quality of services, and equality of access to our services." Next, *Life* staff writer Loudon Wainwright examines the effect of the doctor shortage on one community, Dyersville, Iowa, (population 22,000). This is followed by a critique on the traditional method of educating medical students by doctor and novelist *(The Andromeda Strain)* Michael Crichton. The next excerpt, from a *Wall Street Journal* article by staff reporter Ellen Graham, examines one recent result of the medical care revolution: an increasing number of malpractice suits against doctors. She says that many elderly doctors are retiring earlier out of fear of malpractice suits and that others tend to put patients through batteries of otherwise unnecessary tests in order to protect themselves in the event of a malpractice suit. Dr. Walter Bornemeier, former president of the American Medical Association, gives his prescription for solving the doctor shortage in the next article. Dr. Bornemeier believes that trained paramedics, drawn from the armed forces medical corps and from specially established training programs, can take much of the strain off the doctor. To *Fortune* magazine associate editor Dan Cordtz, this is only a half-way solution. He calls for thorough change from the traditional individual practice of the doctor to greater reliance on group practice. The final selection, from *U.S. News & World Report,* examines the growing influence of electronics in medicine and discusses the potential value of electronic devices in helping to ease the doctor shortage.

WHERE DOCTORS FAIL [1]

In this day of big problems, massively transmitted to an anxious and inflamed citizenry, the American physician has received more than his share of rhetorical abuse. The "in" statement of the avant-garde medical critic is that we in the medical world have developed a "nonsystem, cottage industry" and are populated by a merchant class of greedy Sybarites who subdivide the body according to specialist interest, refuse to make house calls, and preach the gospel

[1] From article by Dr. John H. Knowles, general director of the Massachusetts General Hospital. *Saturday Review.* 53:21-3+. Ag. 22, '70. Copyright 1970 Saturday Review, Inc. Reprinted by permission.

of Puritan asceticism, social Darwinism, and Mark Hanna
—"the public be damned!" Organized medicine—the American Medical Association—emerges as the ogre in the form
of a vast and powerful trade union interested only in the
economic advancement of its members. The medical schools
are not exempt from the avalanche of criticism. Even those
lovely selfless creatures called nurses have been taken to
task for wanting full professionalization through education
and for not spending more time with the patient, or at least
with his back and his bedpan.

The individual patient wants personal, continuous, and
comprehensive care of high quality, and at a reasonable
cost. Interestingly, this is exactly what the physician would
like his patient to have. Both have failed partially for reasons not always under their control. The inexorable expansion of science and technology has resulted in necessary
specialization with attendant discontinuity of care, sub-
division of labor, and increasing costs. What used to be
a one patient - one doctor relationship is now one patient
to one doctor to another doctor to fifteen to twenty people
standing behind each doctor in the hospital and in other
institutions related to health, and the overworked doctor
doesn't like the situation any better than do his patients.

The American doctor continues to enjoy one of the
highest and most respected positions in society, and well
he should. We doctors *do* have much to offer to improve
the quality of people's lives. But we *are* conservative and we
don't want change, and we don't want to face certain facts.

We have failed miserably to meet the public demand
for cost controls and comprehensive health insurance, high
and uniform quality of services, and equality of access to
our services. We have created manpower shortages at all
levels of the health field. We have favored the producers
of health services—hospitals, doctors, and drug companies
—over the consumers of such services.

Our acute, curative, scientific, and technical service is
unexcelled anywhere in the world. Our preventive and

rehabilitative services and our extended care and nursing home facilities are dismal. In other words, high-cost medicine is the best, while low-cost services and those with high benefit-to-cost advantages remain grossly underdeveloped. We have arrived at an "either-or" situation—either we produce or Big Government will muddle in with all its bureaucratic inefficiency and unresponsiveness—and we can look forward to a loss of pluralism, longer coffee breaks, an erosion of individual initiative, and decaying institutions. (Before you write the editor, take a tour through your municipal, state, and Federal hospitals.) I run a voluntary hospital with 6,000 non-civil-service, nonunion employees and 350 private practitioners, and I will pit them against any system of medical care anywhere by any measure—cost, quality, concern, you name it.

We have met the enemy and it is us. Our official organization, the AMA—and I still have my union card—has resisted every major social change in medicine over the past fifty years. It is an incredible track record.

At the turn of the century, the AMA stood at the forefront of progressive thinking and socially responsible action. Its members had been leaders in forming much-needed public health departments in the states during the last half of the nineteenth century. It formed a Council on Medical Education in 1904 and immediately began an investigation of proprietary medical schools. Because of its success in exposing intolerable conditions in those schools, the Carnegie Foundation, at the AMA's request, commissioned Abraham Flexner to study the national scene. His report in 1910 drove proprietary interests out of medical education, established it as a full university function with standards for admission, curriculum development, and clinical teaching. Our present system of medical education, essentially unchanged since the Flexner (and AMA) revolution—and acknowledging its current defects—was accomplished through the work of the AMA. Surely this contribution was and is one of its finest in the public interest. . . .

Starting in 1921, the AMA began its regular opposition to Federal health programs as it fought the Shepard-Towner Act, which provided grants to the states for maternal and child-health programs. It successfully forced President Roosevelt and his advisers away from the inclusion of health insurance in the Social Security Act of 1935. Although it had initially opposed voluntary health insurance, it finally accepted its inevitability and set about to gain complete professional control of its development. Indeed, today the Blue Shield program is largely under the professional control of state and county medical societies.

The major issue besetting the AMA over the past fifty years has been the struggle for the absolute power of self-determination. That is, the autonomy to decide what is best for the profession and what is best for the public, without "outside" interference. Looked at narrowly, the battle pits conservatives against liberals; self-reliant individualists against paternalistic socialists; creative artists against power-hungry bureaucrats. Looked at more broadly, it represents the fears of a proud profession steadily losing power and territory to "others" in the health field. Narrowly, this has been characterized as a battle for money and economic security; more broadly, as a loss of freedom and a reaction to the interposition of outside forces between a doctor and his patient, much as a father resents the interposition of anyone or anything between him and his sons.

The current scene finds the AMA at a rather hostile arm's length from hospitals, medical schools, and the Federal Government and their respective organizations—the American Hospital Association, the Association of American Medical Colleges, and the Department of Health, Education, and Welfare—to say nothing of the American Nurses' Association and the American Public Health Association. The AMA came together briefly with the Association of American Medical Colleges in 1968 to state publicly that there was indeed a critical shortage of physicians—something the AMA had denied steadfastly while lobbying since 1930 against attempts to increase output. But the organization's relationship with these other major national forces in the health field remains cool, to say the least. The situation has degenerated to the point where AMA opposition to any program relating to the nation's health means there must be something good in it for the people. The last great defeat suffered by the AMA was the passage of Medicare in 1965. . . .

I agree that the private sector exercising the initiative of free citizens *can* provide the best solution to regional social issues—but the question remains, will it? My fervent plea is that the AMA seize the opportunity for leadership. Beefing up its public relations department to buy a better image, or spending as much on regressive lobbying as it did against Medicare (nearly $1 million in the first quarter of 1965, a record for any lobby) will not carry the day. Only action will. . . .

Resolution of the mammoth problems besetting the health field demands a holistic, multidisciplinary approach. For example, solving the issues of cost, quality, and equality of access demands fundamental changes in public and private financing mechanisms, public education, manpower supply and use, regional planning, and medical education. The "system" must be changed from the present last-line-of-defense, acute-care, essentially passive approach to one that stresses preventive and rehabilitative services: early detection of disease and keeping people out of hospitals through health education and financial incentives for the producers. At the same time, medicine should be at the forefront on larger issues affecting public health, such as population and pollution control.

The AMA should support compulsory, prepaid health insurance for *all* Americans. It should support standards and quality controls. It should actively stimulate pluralism in medical practice—physicians should be encouraged to join comprehensive, prepaid group practice on a salary-plus-incentive basis. And the AMA should set regional guidelines that will result in restraints on the pricing mechanism for doctors' services. The free-market economy and the tenets of laissez-faire have not, cannot, and will not work for setting physicians' fees. . . .

The AMA does much in the public interest. Its Committee on Alcoholism and Drug Dependence has done a great deal to alert the citizenry and to develop public policy on these two major threats to national health. Similarly, state and county medical societies have seized the initiative in solving obvious problems. Innovations such as the Washington State Medical Society's joint program with medical school interests to develop physician assistants and the Sacramento County, California, Medical Society's CHAP program to strengthen hospital utilization reviews also are noteworthy. We need more of this if the private practice of medicine and our voluntary hospitals are to survive and be strengthened. Let us hope that the progressive spirit underlying these programs will become contagious and that the political and economic muscle of organized medicine can be turned to solving instead of perpetuating the urgent health problems we face.

DILEMMA IN DYERSVILLE [2]

Very desirable opportunity in the U.S.A. for general practitioners and/or group practice. New hospital with latest equipment. Office space available at the hospital. Located in Iowa town of 3-4,000, drawing from an area of 22,000 population in rich farmland with expanding industry. Desirable location for growing family. Good schools locally. Three colleges within 30 miles and universities nearby. Famed Mayo Clinic 100 miles, and 250 miles to Chicago.

This advertisement, published recently in an Irish medical journal, doesn't begin to do justice to the town of Dyersville or to its difficult medical dilemma. . . .

[2] From "Dilemma in Dyersville—Help Wanted: Doctors Needed in a Real Nice Iowa Town With a Brand-New Hospital, Fine Schools and a Future," article by Loudon Wainwright, staff writer. *Life*. 68:48-50+. My. 29, '70. © 1970 Time Inc.

The ad does not really convey the urgency of Dyersville's call for help. The new hospital is a low brick building with a handsome mansard roof which settles comfortably into the hillside on the southwest side of town. The wide expanse of glass is welcoming. Inside the lights are warm, the regulated temperatures perfect, and a walk along the shining corridors reveals spotless rooms in varying, friendly colors. The new equipment in the operating rooms, the delivery room, the emergency rooms and the laboratory positively gleams with its up-to-dateness. More than anything, there's an air about the place, a kind of *readiness*, as if a powerful potential for lifesaving awaited only a call over the public address system.

Yet the $1.7 million hospital, its facilities scarcely used and eighty-nine beds mostly empty, is steadily losing money and may have to close because of the need for doctors, Irish or otherwise, who will bring patients to its facilities. The one local man who staffs the place in every way from patching up automobile accident emergencies to delivering babies to performing gall bladder operations has worked himself close to exhaustion in the year since the hospital opened. The next payment and interest charges on the $750,000 indebtedness come due in July [1970], and the promise that medical help is on the way is quite likely the only thing that will enable the trustees to borrow the money needed to cover current losses. So the citizens of this self-reliant and prosperous community, people who take pride in being good farmers and good managers, are in dead earnest as they offer their town as a good place to work and themselves as good neighbors. . . .

The search for doctors was and continues to be particularly agonizing. A doctor procurement committee has been in touch with hundreds of candidates, sent its members on scouting trips to most of the medical schools and large hospitals in the upper Midwest and even considered a billboard campaign which might seduce a passing physician. When the hospital was completed, an eight-page brochure extolling it and Dyersville as great places for doctors was distributed all over the country. There were few inquiries. The only piece of good fortune occurred when Dr. [Charles A.] Griffin, a year after he left, responded splendidly to a 1,500-signature petition asking him to come home. He resigned from his job in North Carolina, sent the hospital fund a pledge for $5,000 and wrote: "I left Dyersville intending never to return. I shall return intending never to leave."

But the majority of young doctors just had no interest in Dyersville. Trained in various specialties, they didn't want to carry on the sort of general practice that seemed most appropriate in this situation. Instead, they wanted to go to larger communities. A few surgeons nibbled but decided that the shortage of other doctors would have meant too few referrals for surgical work. There were some near things. One man was seriously considering coming to Dyersville, where he was attracted to the rural setting far from the city's crime and clamor. After months of deliberation and suspense, he finally went to a small town in Wisconsin. One ripe candidate went to another town in Iowa. The rejections came hard. "It was like the whole world caved in when they picked another place," Merle Ross [former mayor and one of the hospital's earliest boosters] remembers. "You so want to believe a man's coming that you can't think anything else.". . .

[Since this story appeared in *Life* many doctors asked for more information and the prospects for increasing the hospital staff improved.—Ed.]

"Any doctor who'll come," says Jerome Ungs, one of the town bankers, "will be able to write his own ticket." By that Ungs means that the new doctor will be able to rent office space very cheaply in the Medical Arts Building right next to the hospital, that he will be able to easily get a house mortgage (though at 8 per cent) and even to finance the balance if he hasn't the cash. As it is every place else, inflation is being felt in Dyersville, but the pinch is still slight and a new doctor would quickly be living as well as anyone in town. . . .

The spirit with which the hospital project was tackled provides possibly the most revealing insight into the character of the people who live in Dyersville and around it. Once the community had been convinced of the need for the hospital, hard planning and an urgent drive for funds went ahead in spite of repeated disappointments. When funding goals fell short, businessmen and individuals were asked again and again to increase their pledges. Auctions, entertainments, bake sales, raffles, all were used to raise money, and when it was all done, $900,000 had been pledged. The occasional contribution of local planning, labor and equipment have kept costs down. When an additional piece of wooded property was bought next to the hospital grounds, virtually the whole town turned out with bulldozers, chain saws and axes and cleared out a sizable forest in a single day. The great majority of the people of Dyersville wanted that hospital very badly, and it is going to be little short of a community disaster in pride alone if it cannot be supported.

But all the old-fashioned spirit in the world will not keep the Dyersville Community Hospital operating. Currently about one third of its beds are in use. To meet expenses, twice that number (at $42 a day for a private room, $36 for semiprivate) is necessary. Dr. Griffin, who conducts daily office hours and makes house calls as well as caring for thirty-five or more hospital patients every day, is simply unable to carry a greater load.

It is sad we are in this position [he said recently]. My dream was to see a hospital in Dyersville before I died. I stayed up all night the day we opened to see the sun rise over it. And it's a *good* hospital. The quality of the help is good, the technicians are good. If Charlie Mayo came down here, he wouldn't have any problems. He'd be right at home. The design is so far ahead of its time that with extensions it will be adequate for many years.

Yet only more doctors can bring the hospital to full productivity. And with a U.S. doctor shortage that approaches 50,000, Dyersville's chances are not the best. Of the other men in town, the osteopath is not permitted to practice in the hospital, and the second M.D. chooses to refer his patients to specialists in Dubuque. So Griffin is alone. "I can do 90 per cent of the things my patients present me," he said. "But I'm working more. I used to sleep."

Dr. Griffin caressed the circles under his eyes with his fingers. "The trouble with a lot of doctors these days," he went on, "is that they're doctor-oriented, not patient-oriented; they're more geared to handle their own problems than the patients'. And they don't want sole responsibility either. They want to share the responsibility with someone else."

He leaned back in his chair. "This is where the people live and are," he said. "I came here to serve. We need a guy who wants to come here now, somebody who just wants to take care of the sick."

THE MISEDUCATION OF DOCTORS [3]

A seventeen-year-old who wants to be a doctor faces eleven to fifteen years of training, at a total expense of more than $50,000, before he is ready to begin practice. This extraordinary investment of time and money is one of the most remarkable facts about American medicine. In America, doctors are literally the most educated people we have. The accepted mythology, with its glorification of this extended, expensive training, is that nobody who has the dedication to embark upon such a lengthy program of study could possibly emerge unequipped for the job he had to do.

Yet one can argue that much of medical education is misdirected, and that many physicians are inappropriately trained. If you don't believe this, ask your pediatrician about Jean Piaget [Swiss psychologist specializing in the develop-

[3] Article by Michael Crichton, M.D., author of *The Andromeda Strain* and *Five Patients: The Hospital Explained*. New York *Times*. p 41. O. 16, '70. © 1970 by The New York Times Company. Reprinted by permission.

ment of children's intellectual faculties]—or ask him why he
routinely vaccinates against smallpox. Or ask your internist whom you see yearly why he doesn't do tonometry as
part of your checkup.

How can a person be a student for more than a decade
yet be inadequately trained? The answer lies in a complex
of historical, social, scientific and administrative factors. A
full answer must include both the years of formal training,
and the later refresher courses—or the lack of them—for the
private physician. But central to it all is a single massive
conceptual fallacy: the goal of the doctor-scientist.

Most medical education is inexplicable, except as a program to produce a doctor-scientist. In countries such as
England, there is no foolishness about a doctor-scientist,
and most physicians hold only a B.S. degree; the M.D. is
relatively rare. But in America for the last century, the image
of the clinician-researcher has been increasingly the model,
and it is now central dogma for medical educators, who accept it unquestioningly. Even the public seems to draw a
certain vague satisfaction from thinking that their doctor,
now taking their blood pressure (and in doing so, performing
a job far below his training) could walk out of the office and
into the laboratory, where he would do great things.

In fact, the notion is nonsense. Most M.D.s either go into
research or clinical practice. Few do both—and even fewer
do both well. Every university center has a handful who are
superb, and are widely and justly admired. But to train
every young doctor to be like these men is as foolish as trying
to make every young athlete run 100 yards in under ten
seconds.

Eight years after secondary school, four years after college, the man with an M.D. is neither fish nor fowl: if he
wants to do clinical work, he needs another three to five
years of hospital experience; if he wants to do research, he
probably has to go back to school (or to the National Insti-

tutes) for further training in mathematics and other subjects. One may ask what the student has been doing for all these years. The answer is that he has been working very hard to master subjects, such as the fine points of gross anatomy and organic chemistry, that in later years he will blissfully forget. The doctor-scientist orientation produces a nasty side effect: it takes incoming medical students who are interested in people, and transforms them into doctors interested in diseases. People don't like to be thought of as diseases, as "beautiful cases" of pathology. Medical students who complain about the "dehumanizing influence" of their education are talking about the same thing. Many become psychiatrists by default, since psychiatry seems to be the only warm, human preserve in an otherwise cold, stainless steel, scientific profession.

The practicing doctor, his years of training behind him, makes two disquieting discoveries. First, he finds that he must practice a great deal of unscientific medicine—dealing with the 70 per cent of his patients who have no demonstrable illness, but varying complaints. This calls for behavioral training which he almost certainly lacks. Second, he discovers that his training is rapidly outdated, but the refresher courses run by university doctors are generally abstruse, heavily scientific and lacking the practical details on patient care that he needs. The courses are expensive and a doctor must also accept loss of income from his practice while he is away; many doctors quit going after a few disheartening experiences.

There is great prestige in the idea of the doctor who is also a scientist. It is also fundamentally phony. Even during the Renaissance, there weren't many Renaissance Men, and in a highly complex technical field like medicine, there are even fewer. In the long run the profession will gain greater prestige by training its men appropriately, and abandoning its illusory ideals.

THE DOCTOR AND MALPRACTICE SUITS [4]

"Take two aspirin and call me in the morning."
You don't hear that tired line from doctors much anymore. Nowadays if you phone your family physician and he
suspects any possibility of serious symptoms, he may well
say: "Go straight to the hospital and we'll run you through
a full battery of tests."

Whether your complaint is a headache, a swollen ankle
or chest pains, chances are good your doctor is going to
think twice before he dismisses your case as routine and pre-
scribes nothing more than bed rest.

The reason for this extra caution? Doctors, facing un-
precedented numbers of malpractice suits and sky-high malpractice-insurance rates, freely admit they are practicing
medicine "defensively" these days to guard against potential
suits.

A Prompt Hospital Readmission

Consider, for instance, the case of a Florida housewife
who recently underwent surgery and returned to her doctor
complaining of an infection that developed after the operation. The doctor promptly readmitted her to the hospital
for four days.

"She's doing beautifully," the physician says. "Of course,
she would have recovered just as well at home, but she was
so nervous about the infection, I was afraid she might sue
if something happened and I hadn't taken every precaution."

This year about 10,000 persons are expected to file malpractice suits against doctors. Claims against physicians are
rising 8 per cent to 10 per cent a year. During the past four
years, nationwide increases in malpractice-insurance premiums have averaged 290 per cent, and surgeons in certain
"high-risk" specialties have been hit with much greater increases. Settlements against doctors have occasionally topped
$1 million.

[4] From "Malpractice Suits Rise, Lead Doctors to Treat Patients With Caution," by Ellen Graham, staff reporter, *Wall Street Journal*. p 1+. Ja. 8, '71. Reprinted by permission.

Some insurance companies, saying that they pay out
more in claims than they take in even with higher premiums,
are pulling out of the field of malpractice insurance. Many
physicians are finding it difficult to get coverage at all—
companies have abruptly failed to renew policies in some
states, even though a doctor has never been involved in a suit.

An Air of "Near Hysteria"

"This trend puts physicians in unusually vulnerable positions, creating in some instances an atmosphere of tension
and alarm approaching near hysteria," Eli Bernsweig, the
Department of Health, Education, and Welfare's malpractice specialist, recently told a New York State senate hearing
on malpractice.

The tension is being felt subtly in many areas of patient
care, as doctors act to protect themselves against possible
litigation by ordering more X rays, laboratory studies and
diagnostic tests than ever before. Many doctors insist this
all means better medical care. But often the extra testing
doesn't change the diagnosis or alter the treatment; it merely
serves as expensive ammunition for a doctor to use in court.
And it's the patient of course, who eventually pays for the
longer hospital stays, extra tests and higher doctor bills.
(Some doctors say they have raised their fees as much as 20
per cent during the past year to cover their higher insurance costs.)

Just how many extra lab tests and days in the hospital
are being fostered by this fear of malpractice is impossible
to determine. For one thing, few doctors are willing to con-
cede, at least publicly, that such fear is their motive for ordering an additional blood test or an X ray. And hospital committees that watch for overuse of hospital rooms, as well as
health-insurance companies that scrutinize claims looking
for unnecessary procedures, term it impossible to tell
whether a doctor ordered a test on the basis of sound medical
judgment or to avoid a malpractice suit.

Fearing Errors of Omission

"Many doctors will order procedures that actually they feel aren't necessary—tests they wouldn't order on their own family—but they're afraid of omitting a test or a detail which might be held against them in case of a later suit," says Dr. Carl A. Hoffman, chairman of the American Medical Association's professional-liability committee.

A New York physician adds, "You can often make a diagnosis with a minimum number of tests. Now we do extra tests to confirm the diagnosis. For instance, if a patient comes in with a swollen ankle and I'm 99 per cent sure it's just sprained, I'll take an X ray anyway to make certain it isn't broken or fractured. A few years ago, I would have taken that 1 per cent chance it wasn't a fracture."

Just how these extra procedures can increase medical costs is described by a Florida gynecologist who says doctors in his part of the country are now doing routine D&Cs (dilation and curettage, or scraping of the uterus) on every miscarriage patient. There's a remote chance of complications if the procedure is omitted.

"Only about one third of the patients actually need D&Cs," he says. "But there have been a few suits over this issue, and we aren't taking any chances." He says the extra surgery and hospitalization for the D&C raise the cost of a miscarriage to $275 from about $50.

Partially to keep pace with the workload produced when supercautious doctors order more tests, hospitals report they are beefing up X-ray and laboratory crews and ordering new equipment—which is an expensive process.

And hospital labs aren't the only facilities where the squeeze is on. Beds are in short supply because doctors are becoming increasingly quick to admit and slow to discharge patients. Many of these hospital admissions are patients who require minor surgery—surgery that used to be done in a doctor's office.

"A couple of years ago, I'd take off cysts in my office," says one Los Angeles general practitioner. "Now if I have to do any surgery, I send patients to the hospital. Of course, this adds to the cost of medical care."

Once a patient is in the hospital, chances are good he will stay longer because doctors want to keep patients under careful supervision in case of unforeseen complications. As one doctor said in an AMA survey, "If you're practicing medicine, the law is looking over your shoulder." He says sometimes even if he wants to discharge a patient from the hospital, he will keep him in a few days longer to avoid "repercussions."

But many physicians argue that all these precautions add up to better care.

"Much better treatment is being given in emergency rooms today because of the malpractice scare," says Dr. Cyril Wecht, president of the American College of Legal Medicine. "The tests cost more, but we're saving more lives."

Because of its tense and impersonal atmosphere, the hospital emergency room has been a source of numerous lawsuits. Patients are more likely to sue a doctor they don't know, and the risk of error increases in emergency rooms, where doctors are subjected to heavy tension and are susceptible to mounting fatigue.

Dr. Wecht maintains that some of this risk has been eliminated because emergency-room patients now get more extensive testing and are more often admitted to the hospital for observation. As an example, he says patients complaining of chest pains are given electrocardiograms more routinely now. Too often in the past, he adds, untested patients were discharged, only to die a few hours later of heart attacks.

"Sure, the extra tests are expensive," says Dr. Wecht. "But what's medicine all about? Is it to see how few dollars we spend and ignore how many lives are lost with a penny-pinching approach?"

The other side of the coin, however, is that some doctors have begun to shun risky procedures or new, untried treatments because of the possible legal consequences if the methods should backfire.

"Doctors have been painted into the corner of doing what will keep us out of trouble rather than what's necessarily best for the patient," says Dr. William F. Quinn, a Los Angeles surgeon.

And the regents of the American College of Surgeons recently warned, "Instead of attempting procedures which may cure the patient but have a higher risk of failure and exposure to the threat of a lawsuit, some surgeons may prefer to use standard, proved, conservative methods which might bring relief to the patient but will not cure him."

The San Diego County (California) Medical Society surveyed its members last year on the question of malpractice and how it had affected their treatment of patients. Of about 1,000 doctors responding, more than 350 said the fear of a malpractice suit had caused them to stop performing certain duties or stop using particular procedures. Some doctors, for instance, said they gave up emergency-room duty. Others stopped doing orthopedic and other types of surgery. Still others said they no longer would administer an anesthetic. And some even refused to perform tonsillectomies.

A New York anesthesiologist, noting the high incidence of suits and large damage awards resulting from spinal-anesthetic mishaps, confesses, "If I have the choice between a spinal and a general anesthetic, I'll frequently choose a general—even though a spinal is, on the whole, safer."

Surgeons are perhaps the most frequent targets for litigation. One, on New York's Long Island, says that if he was performing an appendectomy and discovered an abdominal tumor, he wouldn't touch the tumor until he had first sewn up the patient, brought him out of anesthesia and obtained his signed consent to perform the necessary additional surgery. Result: Increased risk for the patient and added medical costs.

Some doctors try to ward off lawsuits by refusing to prescribe certain drugs with many side effects. Dr. Samuel Horowitz, a Los Angeles general practitioner, decided two years ago to stop prescribing birth-control pills. Instead, he refers patients to a nearby family planning clinic.

Still others resort to more frequent consultations to verify their own diagnoses. "A doctor's greatest comfort during a suit is knowing that a colleague was consulted," says one doctor. Dr. William Quinn of Los Angeles agrees. "Just the other day I saw a patient who needed breast surgery. Since she also had a heart condition, I had to call in a heart specialist to confirm that she'd be a reasonable risk for surgery. It's important to have his statement on the record, but it cost the patient an extra consultation fee."

Even one malpractice suit in a community is enough to make doctors jittery. A doctor in Orlando, Florida, was recently sued successfully for $89,000 when a woman died after complications that arose during childbirth. The suit shook the medical profession there.

"We're more cautious in delivering babies now," says Dr. Robert T. Hoover, an Orlando obstetrician, adding that he is more likely to do cesarean deliveries than in the past.

"If I don't think a patient can deliver normally, a cesarean is a good out, rather than face the possibility of complications." Dr. Hoover says two Orlando physicians eliminated obstetrics from their practices after the uproar over the suit.

"There's a big risk in obstetrics," he says. "In this day of modern medicine, the mother and baby are expected to survive. If they don't, the first one blamed is the doctor." He adds that in cases of maternal death in childbirth, the doctor has a 50-50 chance of being sued, regardless of the cause of death.

Besides inhibiting doctors in their treatment of high-risk cases, the fear of malpractice and the dissolving insurance market may be taking its toll in other ways—specifically, the availability of medical care in some areas.

In Utah, for example, young doctors have found it difficult to get malpractice insurance unless they join a group practice that is already covered—and most of these are in cities.

"Our small towns are finding it hard to replace a doctor who dies or retires because young doctors can't practice solo anymore," says Dr. Chester B. Powell, a Salt Lake City neurosurgeon and head of the Utah Medical Society's medical-legal council.

There are also indications that states with especially high malpractice-insurance rates are finding it harder and harder to attract new doctors or even hold on to well-established physicians.

A young neurosurgeon may think twice before shelling out nearly $5,000 a year for adequate coverage in California, for instance, if he can settle down in New Hampshire instead and pay about $325 for the same policy. Older doctors tapering off their practices have sometimes found that their volume of work doesn't justify continuing a practice at high insurance rates. They've begun to choose early retirement instead.

Rx FOR THE FAMILY DOCTOR SHORTAGE [5]

The most serious health problem facing our nation today is the shortage of family doctors—the general practitioners, pediatricians and internists who provide the bulk of what we call primary care. Forty years ago, we had one such doctor for each 1,139 people. Today we have only one for each 1,750.

The symptoms of the spreading shortage are everywhere obvious: in the increasing difficulty in finding a doctor at night or on weekends; in the way middle-class patients now queue up at the charity clinics and emergency rooms of our hospitals; in the lengthening delays in obtaining appointments for routine care.

[5] From article by Dr. Walter C. Bornemeier, former president, American Medical Association. *Reader's Digest*. 97:103-7. Jl. '70. Reprinted by permission.

None of this happens because we doctors want it that way. It's simply that the demand for all medical services—fed by ever-wider hospitalization and surgical insurance, and by such Government plans as Medicare and Medicaid—is constantly running ahead of the supply of doctors. From 1958 to 1968, national spending for personal health services soared from $12.8 billion to $57.1 billion. We're now spending 6.5 per cent of our gross national product on health; by 1975, this figure is expected to rise to 10 per cent. Moreover, the imbalance between supply and demand cannot be solved simply by opening the throttle on the nation's 101 medical colleges. For one thing, so many of our graduating doctors now go into specialties, research, teaching, public health and industrial medicine that only 38 per cent of our present physicians can be classified as family doctors. For another, a medical education now takes so long (usually eight years) that even doubling the entering class of medical students, beginning next fall, would add only 30,000 doctors to the total turned out by the medical schools in the next ten years. This number would not even cover the shortage currently predicted for 1975!

Neglected Resources

The American Medical Association, which represents the vast majority of practicing physicians in the United States, believes there is something we can do—right away—that will begin to relieve the shortage of family doctors. We of the AMA believe that doing it will make working conditions for family doctors more attractive and eventually draw more doctors into this vital field. Also, our solution will not require major legislation or huge appropriations. And we are certain that it will result in better care for more people at a lower unit cost.

What we advocate is simply that private physicians begin immediately to divest themselves of all routine functions that can be performed by assistants and associates, who will spend the bulk of their training time working in doctors' offices. This is not at all revolutionary. Until fifty years ago, doctors in this country trained by working in the offices of established physicians. And even with the rise of the university-affiliated medical colleges, we doctors continued to train the bulk of our nonprofessional nurses and office technicians.

Where will the pool of high-grade medical workers to be thus upgraded come from? We have in this country two conspicuously wasted resources. First, there are at least 285,000 inactive registered nurses. After marrying and getting their families started, thousands of them would be delighted to come back into medicine with the higher pay and status of a doctor's assistant.

In addition, our armed services each year discharge more than 30,000 medically trained personnel. These men have received several hundred hours of medical instruction at an estimated cost to the taxpayer of up to $25,000. Perhaps 5,000 of them have been qualified for "independent duty," meaning that they could go out on a long submarine cruise as the only medical man aboard, or could look after servicemen at an isolated radar station. Other good prospects are those who have manned front-line medical stations in Vietnam. Yet, up to now, virtually the only civilian medical career open to these men—even after twenty years' service—has been that of hospital orderly.

Putting these retired nurses and former corpsmen to work in doctors' offices would dramatically increase the availability and accessibility of private health care in this country. It would also apply a needed brake to health costs, which are rising at twice the rate of inflation. And I am not speculating about things that might be. I'm describing changes in private medical practice which have already become a reality under some thirty physician's-assistant programs initiated in the United States over the past five years. Some examples:

Medex

In Seattle, the University of Washington Medical School and the Washington State Medical Association's Education and Research Foundation have set up a program to train former medical corpsmen, who are brought into Seattle for a three-month brush-up course on civilian medical procedures. After graduation, these Medex (from the French term, *médecin extension*—literally, "physician extension") are sent out across the state to work in the offices of doctors who agree to act as their preceptors and to employ them at salaries ranging from $8,000 to $12,000 a year after twelve months of on-the-job training. (While learning they receive $500 and up a month.)

The first fourteen Medex are now on the job and sharply boosting doctor productivity and morale. Dr. Wilfred Gamon, a general practitioner in Cheney and a member of the state board of medical examiners, is as proud as a father of his Medex, Bob Woodruff, who assists a staff physician at the Eastern Washington State College infirmary, which Dr. Gamon and his partners handle on contract as part of their new medical center. When not looking after the routine health problems of the 6,000 students, Medex Woodruff, a handsome ex-Green Beret who looks like a college student himself, pitches in with Dr. Gamon's private patients.

At first, Dr. Gamon asked each of these patients whether he objected. Then one of them quietly reminded him, "I trusted somebody like your Medex with the life of my son." With the help of Medex Woodruff, Dr. Gamon and his partners feel that they are now turning out about 25 per cent more work. "Without Bob," Dr. Gamon says, "we would be overwhelmed."

Other Washington doctors are equally pleased with their Medex. Dr. Jesse Sewell, forty-three, had been trying to provide medical care over several thousand square miles of sparsely settled wheatlands in central Washington by driving hundreds of miles a week and occasionally flying his own

plane on emergency calls. Finally, hospitalized after a colli-
sion with a snowplow during a blizzard, he had almost decided to give up his practice as too strenuous. Instead, he
visited Fairchild Air Force Base and interested retiring corpsmen Louis Lebert and Oren Kent in becoming Medex.

Six months later, with one Medex stationed in Odessa
and the other in Harrington, Dr. Sewell had doubled the
number of patients he was caring for and was being peti-
tioned by the people of another town to open a third office
in their community. He has been delighted with the competence of his two assistants. On his first day, Medex Kent
picked up a heart murmur in a 220-pound high-school foot-
ball lineman, and soon after that Medex Lebert found a hair-
line fracture that both the hospital radiologist and Dr. Sewell
had missed. Summing up happily, Dr. Sewell says, "For the
first time since I got out of medical school, I'm practicing the
kind of medicine I dreamed of when I was a student.' . . .

Problems That Might Arise

As with every program of medical reform, there are questions. Is it legal, for example, for doctors to delegate functions?

The laws of all fifty states give a physician broad and unlimited powers to delegate tasks to others so long as appropriate training has been given, the work is performed com-
petently and the tasks are performed under the doctor's
direction. This direction may be over the shoulder, by phone,
or under standing instructions and subject to the doctor's
later review.

Are there insurance liability problems?

The bulk of malpractice suits involve anesthesiology in
hospitals; none of the physician's-assistant programs described are in this field. Most alumni of current physician's-
assistant programs have had little difficulty in obtaining insurance coverage at nominal rates.

Will patients feel they are getting second-class treatment? . . .

Studies show that this is sometimes the reaction of low-income patients and of the very rich. Persons in the middle-income brackets, who are the chief support of private doctors, realize that having an assistant work with the doctor can only help to improve the overall quantity and quality of medical care.

Does the creation of physician's assistants mean we can let up on the pressure to produce more and better doctors?

Not at all. Obviously, we must have many more doctors as well as many more doctor's assistants if we are going to avoid a further crisis. But this will take some basic and time-consuming reforms in our system of medical education. Personally, I think the time is past when we can spend so much time on training that we keep a would-be doctor economically dependent and nonproductive until he is almost thirty.

CHANGE BEGINS IN THE DOCTOR'S OFFICE [6]

When Dr. Sidney Lee, associate dean for hospital programs at Harvard Medical School, is asked what is wrong with American medicine, he has a prompt and characteristically blunt answer: "Doctors!" He has a good point. The nation's 313,000 active physicians are quite properly the main target for the critics of the health care system. The doctor created the system. They run it. And they are the most formidable obstacle to its improvement. It is the doctor who decides which patients will be treated, where, under what conditions, and for what fee; who will enter the hospital, for what therapy, and for how long; what drugs will be purchased and in what quantities. The United States alone among the world's developed countries has given the medical fraternity such freedom. The profession not only can, but should, be held accountable for the way it uses its power.

[6] From article by Dan Cordtz, associate editor. Fortune. 81:84-9+. Ja. '70. Courtesy of Fortune Magazine.

The trouble with doctors is not that they are more avaricious than other people. Indeed, many of them are dedicated men, who work hard for their high incomes. The real charge against them is that they have been short-sighted, timid, and far too slow to recognize and adapt to change. Only recently did the leaders of organized medicine reluctantly recognize the fact that Americans regard decent health care as one of their rights—not a privilege, or a commodity to be sold by medical men in the open market. Motivated by groundless fears of oversupply, doctors have discouraged the expansion of their own ranks, until now they must acknowledge a serious shortage. Even if every effort were made, that shortage could not be alleviated for at least the next decade. Yet most doctors, far from taking the lead, continue to resist innovations aimed at making the health care system more efficient and responsive to public needs. . . .

Much more is involved in the nation's health, of course, than medical services. Environment, mores, and genetics also play large roles. And more is involved in the supply of medical services than the number of physicians. But their availability is extremely important, not only to the adequacy of care but particularly to perception of its adequacy. . . .

Since 1950, the number of physicians has grown about 25 per cent faster than total population, and that margin is expected to increase as medical schools belatedly open their doors wider. But such overall figures conceal some trends that have important implications for the availability of care. In recent years many doctors have turned away from patient care to work in research laboratories, industry, public health, and other institutions, to teach, or to serve as hospital administrators—all functions of great importance for the future. One third of all doctors now devote themselves to such activities. As a consequence, the number of M.D.s caring for private patients actually declined 10 per cent relative to population between 1950 and 1965—to 92 for each 100,000 Americans. Specialization took a further toll. The doctor-patient ratio of those providing family care (general practitioners, internists, and pediatricians) fell by one third—to 50 per 100,000. (In the 1930s, when almost all doctors were in patient care and 70 per cent were general practitioners, a ratio of 135 per 100,000 was regarded as desirable.)

Where the System Fails

The most glaring shortcoming of the system is the unavailability of care to the poor, the isolated, and members of minority groups. . . . [But] the poor and the isolated are by no means the only ones dismayed and discontented by the way medical costs are now being distributed. Anger about medical costs and the inconvenience and impersonality of care is spreading among the majority of middle-class Americans. Given the fact that the shortage of doctors is going to continue, the medical profession must find ways to improve its productivity. Most critics have centered their attention on three potentially fruitful ways to accomplish this: more extensive use of professionals who are not M.D.s, expansion of group practice, and broad-scale application of computer systems and other new technologies.

Technological innovations hold considerable promise. Duke University's Department of Community Health Sciences is doing research that may provide practicing physicians with the advantages of data processing in making patient-care decisions. The department sees as feasible such improvements as a computer-stored data bank of diagnostic information wired to a terminal located conveniently close to the doctor, enabling him speedily to check his diagnosis of a particular illness with the computer's data about the illness in question.

Duke has also pioneered in the so-called "multiphasic screening clinics," which are now in operation in fourteen locations across the country. As the Commonwealth Fund describes its operation, "This unit will conduct chemical and electronic tests necessary for physical examination. Since much of the equipment can now be automated, it can be operated by technicians and can process both patients and the clinical data collected on them very rapidly. Through the screening clinic, the physician, at no expenditure of his own time, can obtain an important clinical-information profile on his patient." Other uses of electronic equipment include two-way television hookups between hospitals and outlying field stations manned by nurses. One now links a medical station at Boston's Logan Airport with Massachusetts General Hospital.

Cutting Down on the Bookkeeping

Group practice, if the group is of sufficient size, can relieve the physician of almost all of his nonmedical burdens. John R. Johnson, executive administrator of the Palo Alto Medical Clinic, estimates that the average doctor in private practice spends more than 25 per cent of his time on business (bookkeeping, billing, ordering supplies, etc.). "If a doctor uses us right," he says, "he can reduce that to 1 per cent." Economies of scale can also enable groups to provide time-saving in-house laboratory facilities and equipment. And group practice gives the doctor and his patient ready access to specialists in other fields. In spite of these advantages, however, only 12 per cent of all practicing private physicians engage in any kind of group practice; just half of them are full-time members of comprehensive multispecialty groups. Many medical students express an intention to enter group practice, but the percentage of doctors doing so is not increasing much right now.

Part of the reason is money. Salaries for members of a group are usually well under what a hustling physician can earn on his own. Dr. John Knowles, director of Massachusetts General Hospital, tells of a large western group that is trying to recruit an orthopedic surgeon at a salary of $40,000—with no takers. "An orthopedic surgeon can easily make $80,000 a year on his own," Dr. Knowles explains. Further, a doctor just starting out may be reluctant to join a group because there are so few of them. If he finds his associates uncongenial, he may not be able to locate another. He will then have to launch his own practice after having wasted several years.

Splitting Up the Job

"Health care teams" offer the brightest opportunity for improvement of productivity. At present, because of the wide gap between their education and that of others in the medical field, doctors routinely perform many tasks that are beneath their level of competence. Many of them could be handled better by persons trained less broadly but more intensively. If large numbers of such functional specialists were available, physicians could work largely as team leaders—keeping for themselves only the duties demanding the highest skills. Other members of the team, working independently or under the supervision of doctors, would be assigned responsibility commensurate with their education and training.

The mechanics of this eminently sensible idea are difficult to work out. What is required first of all is a detailed analysis of all the duties involved in caring for various types of patients. These must be evaluated in terms of their critical nature, and the kind and degree of skill required to carry out each. They must be divided up in some rational way. Then educational and training programs must be designed, and candidates recruited by the attractions of good salaries and opportunities for advancement. Doctors must be persuaded to use such assistants fully. (The history of physician-nurse relationships is not encouraging on this point.) Finally, and perhaps most difficult of all, medical licensing laws must be changed, and common standards established across the country.

Many schools have already launched experimental programs to train a variety of people in services related to health care. Several are training a new category, the "physician's assistant," who will perform an array of routine chores—

measuring, testing, and giving therapy—that now consume much of the doctor's time and energy. At Duke University School of Medicine, and at the University of Washington School of Medicine in Seattle, the courses of training, which do not lead to a degree, are designed for persons with some previous medical experience, most of whom are medical corpsmen returning from military service. Another school, Alderson-Broaddus College in Philippi, West Virginia, has just started a four-year baccalaureate program that will recruit students directly from high school.

Twenty-nine students have already finished their two-year course at Duke. Dr. D. Robert Howard, director of the program, says that each graduate had more than a dozen job offers. The University of Washington took in its first fifteen students last June for a three-month crash course. After classroom work in the subjects where the men were least experienced—psychiatry, pediatrics, geriatrics, and chronic disease—they were placed in doctors' offices for on-the-job training. All fifteen are now working in rural areas where physicians are most hard-pressed.

The Need for Supporting Troops

Ultimately, however, the future of the health care team concept will depend on the willingness of doctors to accept and utilize paramedical personnel. The numbers of such people have been minuscule thus far, and most have been trained in areas of severe shortage. If their numbers grow rapidly, the early enthusiasm for them may dwindle. Already, a local medical society in California has brought charges of practicing medicine without a license against a neurosurgeon's assistant who—under instructions—removed stitches from a patient's incision.

The attitudes of the doctors may be based on fear of competition. But it is also true that patients themselves may resent being handed over to assistants. Obstetricians are probably the most overtrained, underutilized doctors in the whole profession. Only a tiny number of births involve the kind of complications for which they train so arduously. But it is still difficult to visualize large numbers of middle-class women voluntarily forgoing the comforting presence of an obstetrician at the maternal bedside.

Doctors also resist the kind of reorganization that health teams would require out of a genuine concern for the quality of care. But many members of the profession express reservations about the quality that the present primitive system delivers. "Medical care in the United States," declares Dr. Jacobus Potter, associate dean of New York University School of Medicine, "is like the little girl with the little curl in the middle of her forehead. When it's good, it's the best anywhere. When it's bad, it's appalling."

WILL ELECTRONICS SOLVE THE
DOCTOR SHORTAGE? [7]

Reprinted from *U.S. News & World Report.*

Chalk up fresh gains for one of this country's most promising new industries—the rapidly growing field of "medical electronics."

The name sounds complicated. But it refers basically to two things:

Computers, and equipment linked to them, for medical examinations, diagnosis and treatment.

Other electronic devices that are widening skills and capabilities of the best-trained physicians and surgeons.

For doctors and patients, the array of sophisticated products promises revolutionary changes in the cost and quality of health care.

In many instances, the new developments are credited with saving or extending human lives in ways that would have been impossible a few years ago.

[7] From article in *U.S. News & World Report.* 68:87-9. Je. 15, '70.

Miracles of Science

For a random sampling of what is happening—

Under the Kaiser Foundation Medical Care Program in California, members of a health care plan pay less than $3.50 for a complete, automated physical examination which includes 50 tests and takes two to three hours. A physician, at a later appointment, evaluates the data and explains the results.

At the University of Texas Southwestern medical school in Dallas, a computer hooked up to a TV set tests vision by mapping eye movements. A variation from the normal pattern can detect the presence of a disease affecting eyesight.

A physician at Massachusetts General Hospital, Boston, can sit in a "telediagnosis" room and examine, by using television, an injured person in the medical station at Boston's Logan Airport, several miles distant.

A new blood analyzer, the Auto-Chemist, can handle as many as 135 separate blood samples per hour, and make twenty-four different measurements on each. The cost, per twenty-four tests: about $8.

More than 40,000 Americans now wear electronic pacemakers to regulate their heartbeats. On the way: a nuclear-powered mechanical heart that can be implanted in a patient's chest.

A battery-operated reading aid for the blind permits sightless persons to read newspapers, magazines and other printed material through vibrations against a fingertip. Still in the experimental stage—but designed for eventual large-scale production—the device was developed by a Stanford University professor whose teen-age daughter is blind.

Lasers—concentrated beams of light—are being used almost routinely in eye operations to weld detached retinas.

Latest hearing aids are so tiny they are almost invisible, thanks to progress in miniaturizing batteries.

These and scores of other innovations are part of the
swing toward putting science and technology to work in
creasingly in medical care.

Welcome Advances

The changes come none too soon, in the view of health
care authorities.

Costs of medical services—including fees of physicians
surgeons and dentists, hospital bills, and hospital and sur
gical insurance—have zoomed at twice the rate of other price
in the past five years. . . .

Shortages of doctors, nurses and medical technicians are
increasing at the very time demand for wider health protec
tion is rising. . . .

More and more hospitals are installing monitoring de
vices that permit a nurse at a single console to keep tabs or
several patients at once, watching their blood pressure, tem
perature, heartbeat and breathing rate.

Computer-aided diagnosis of mental illness is being tested
in Rockford, Illinois, at the H. Douglas Singer Zone Center
a new mental-health facility established by the state.

A three-minute, computer-based breathing test to aid in
early detection of crippling lung diseases has been developed
at the University of Nebraska, and a miniature system cap
able of spotting the early-warning signs of a heart attack ha
been developed by Smith Kline Instruments, Inc., of Palo
Alto, California.

Hospitals in four Ohio cities are tied into a computer
center at Ohio State University's college of medicine. Physi
cians at each of the hospitals can query the computer about
latest medications and treatments for a particular disease.

Now computers are moving into the area of disease pre
vention. They are being put to use increasingly in "multi
phasic" physical exams, aimed at spotting danger signals of
diseases or abnormalities that otherwise might go undetected

An individual begins his computerized health checkup
by marking a stack of punched cards or a machine-readable

questionnaire. Then he moves on to a battery of physiological tests and X rays. The whole process takes no more than
an hour or two, and can be done by nurses or medical technicians.

The test results are fed into the computer and compared
with results that are normal for a large segment of the population. If a patient's report varies from this pattern, or indicates any unusual symptoms, a physician can make more
detailed tests. . . .

A Few Snags

While the outlook for electronics in health care is for
large-scale expansion in days to come, the field is not without
its problems.

For one thing, much of the complicated equipment, especially for hospital use, is made to order. Thus the cost is
not as low as it might be if the equipment could be bought
"off the shelf." Repair and maintenance costs are steep.

Medical experts say there is a shortage of technicians
trained to operate complex devices. Many hospitals now find
it essential to add an electronics engineer or two to their
staffs. Physicians are having to take courses in machine operation and learn to interpret results.

Complaints have arisen among some medical men about
lack of standards or controls to protect physicians and patients from shoddy workmanship or safety hazards in the
operation of the new equipment.

Still, the necessity for lightening the mounting burden of
medical care is so great that computers and electronic machines inevitably will be needed in increasing numbers to
supplement human attention, health authorities point out.

From Carter F. Henderson, New York management consultant, comes this observation:

Consider that there are about 10,000 known diseases, 100,000
observable findings, and anywhere from 10,000 to 100,000 available treatments.

Add to that the fact that new medical knowledge is growing at a prodigious rate—so fast that the 1970 medical-school graduate may find that 90 per cent of his resources for observation and treatment are outmoded by the time he reaches age forty-five.

All this suggests the reason why the computer and allied technical equipment are on the way to becoming the physician's best friend, and chief assistant in the practice of medicine.

III. NATIONAL HEALTH INSURANCE:
DO WE NEED IT?

III. NATIONAL HEALTH INSURANCE: DO WE NEED IT?

EDITOR'S INTRODUCTION

According to the U.S. Health Insurance Institute, about 170 million Americans have some form of insurance against hospitalization and about 130 million Americans are insured against regular medical expenses. These are impressive figures, but turn them around and they tell a different story. Fully 35 million Americans, 15 per cent of the population, have no insurance whatever against the crushing expense of hospitalization (which often may be more than $100 a day in urban hospitals) and another 75 million Americans are not insured against the expenses incurred in any extended illness. Insurance companies paid out $7 billion in claims in 1970 for hospital expenses of policy holders. However this was only a bit more than half the hospital bills incurred by Americans in 1970. Another $6 billion more came out of the pockets of individual Americans to pay their hospital bills.

Even before the massive increase in health costs became a national issue in the late 1960s and early 1970s, Congress was considering proposals for national health insurance. As far back as 1948, President Harry S. Truman proposed a national health insurance program. Nothing ever came of it, mainly because of the powerful opposition of organized medicine which denounced health insurance as socialized medicine.

As health costs began to spiral, the issue again gained public prominence. In 1966 Congress passed legislation establishing health insurance for the two groups most heavily affected by the expenses of medical care: the elderly (Medicare) and the poor (Medicaid). The majority of Americans—those nonelderly and nonindigent—were not protected by either Medicare or Medicaid. Should they be covered? This section is concerned with that controversial issue.

The first selection, from *U.S. News & World Report*, surveys the background of the controversy and describes the various national health insurance plans that have been introduced in Congress. The next two selections, by medical affairs writers, deal with Medicare and Medicaid. The first of these, by Fred Anderson, staff associate of the National Academy of Engineering, describes the workings of the two programs. The second, by Irvin Block, describes some of the deficiencies of the programs. There follows an excerpt from *Business Week*, describing how national health insurance works in Britain, Canada, and Sweden. The next two articles discuss whether national health insurance is either needed or feasible. Rashi Fein, professor of the economics of medicine at Harvard University, argues the affirmative; Dr. Paul Ashton, president of the California Professional Guild, the negative. Then President Richard M. Nixon outlines his plan for Health Maintenance Organizations—a new form of group insurance for comprehensive care, supported by both government and private funds. This plan owes something to the prepaid group practice plans described in the final selection from *Fortune* magazine.

HEALTH CARE FOR ALL: WHO WILL PAY THE BILL? [1]

Reprinted from *U.S. News & World Report*.

Clamor about rising medical costs is about to bring major changes in this contry's health care system.

Conviction is growing that before long—perhaps in two or three years—the United States will adopt a national health insurance program covering everyone, regardless of ability to pay.

[1] From "Prepaid Medical Care For All—When . . . Who'll Pay the Bill." *U.S. News & World Report*. 69:26-9. Ag. 10, 70.

"We're going to have it, no question about that," says an insurance company executive. "It's mainly a matter of working out the details." . . .

Already moves are afoot in this direction. At least five broad plans for overhauling the present health care system are up for study. Three have been introduced in Congress. Others are on the way. Each has the aim of assuring medical and hospital care for anyone who needs it. . . .

As yet, all of these are tentative, subject to revision. Nobody really knows how much an across-the-board health plan would cost, how it would be paid for or whether it could be made to work.

The plans advanced thus far differ in financing, in method of operation and in degree of reliance on the private health insurance structure.

An Area of Agreement

On one point, however, there is no disagreement. That is the recognition that paying bills is only part of the health care problem. Just as important, say medical authorities, is how to deliver the benefits that people want and need.

Experience the past few years with the Federal Medicare program for the elderly, and with the Medicaid program for the needy—now costing taxpayers about $14 billion a year, all told—has shown that merely underwriting payments is not enough.

Ways must be found to provide more physicians, nurses and technicians, and more hospital and clinical facilities.

"We have learned, I hope, that simply pouring billions of dollars into a system that is already overstrained won't work," says Dr. Russell B. Roth. An Erie, Pennsylvania, urologist, he is speaker of the American Medical Association's house of delegates.

A Plan for All

Latest official sign of the swing toward universal health care came in a White House task-force report submitted to President Nixon on June 30 [1970].

The report said that "all consumers should have access to health care without hardship or humiliation and, as far as possible, with some voice in how it is planned and some choice of how it is furnished."

Walter J. McNerney, president of the Blue Cross Association, who headed the task force, declared: "The time is right for action."

Others in the medical field and in Government appear to share that view. . . .

A wide range of individuals and groups are involved in current moves toward national health insurance. For example:

> Labor unions are pushing for greater benefits in contracts with management, to safeguard workers against rising medical expenses.
>
> Companies are upset over the inflationary impact of health assistance in their operating costs.
>
> General Motors Corporation notes:
>
> "For the twelve-month period starting October 1, 1970, the increased cost nationwide for unchanged GM hospital-surgical-medical and drug expense coverages will be about $67 million, a 25 per cent increase over the current level of costs."
>
> General Electric Company reports that for the years 1965 through 1969, a period when people on its payroll increased by 24 per cent, health care expenses rose by more than 81 per cent.
>
> Insurance companies are concerned about rising premiums and the prospect that more and more people will be priced out of the market for private health policies.
>
> According to the Health Insurance Institute, while 176 million individuals have some form of private health insurance, another 30 million have no coverage at all. Many who do own policies

find they do not provide enough money to pay the costs of a long or expensive illness.

Traditionally conservative physicians' groups, including the American Medical Association, are moving in the direction of a partial Federal subsidy for health care, despite worries that broader Government controls may be involved.

Public health administrators claim the present method of providing medical services is "outworn, expensive and outrageously inefficient." Many of these officials see a national insurance system as one way to bring about more-efficient use of health care resources.

Using Private Firms

Two of the broad plans under discussion—one proposed by Aetna Life & Casualty, another by the AMA—would draw to a large extent on the capabilities of the private health insurance companies. People of some means would pay for their health care benefits, as at present. The poor, and others unable to qualify for insurance, would get free benefits paid for by Government.

A bill embodying the AMA's proposals was introduced in Congress on July 21 by Representatives Richard Fulton (Democrat), of Tennessee, and Joel Broyhill (Republican), of Virginia.

Two additional plans—one backed by the AFL-CIO, the second sponsored by the Committee for National Health Insurance—would, in effect, provide compulsory health insurance for the entire population, paid for by Federal taxes.

Representative Martha Griffiths (Democrat), of Michigan, has introduced a bill that would carry out many of the AFL-CIO proposals.

Senator Edward Kennedy (Democrat), of Massachusetts, has indicated that he will sponsor in the Senate the plan worked out by the Committee for National Health Insurance. This group was headed by the late Walter Reuther, president of the United Auto Workers Union, a persistent critic of the present health care system. After Mr. Reuther's death a few months ago, leadership of the committee was taken over by Leonard Woodcock, his successor at the UAW.

Still another plan for universal health insurance, put forward by Senator Jacob Javits (Republican), of New York, and introduced in the Senate on April 14 [1970], would depend heavily on taxes to pay physicians' and hospital bills. But the plan would leave a role for private insurers to provide some benefits for individuals who could afford them.

The price tags for all these proposals are vague. Estimates of the annual cost of providing health insurance for everyone in the United States range between $15 billion and $40 billion a year.

Backers of the plans that would draw on the machinery of the private insurance industry say their proposals would be less expensive than turning the job over to the Federal Government.

Proponents of programs to be supported entirely by taxes say such public financing is the only way to guarantee that medical and hospital care will be available for everyone.

A Long History

Efforts to provide some form of universal prepaid health care go back a long way.

In November 1945, President Harry S. Truman sent Congress a special message calling for a comprehensive medical insurance plan for people of all ages. It was to be financed by a rise of 4 per cent in Social Security taxes.

The Truman idea stirred a storm of controversy centering on the issue of "socialized medicine," and was never pushed in Congress.

In 1965, Congress added two amendments to the Social Security program. One established Medicare, a Federal program of hospital insurance for nearly all people aged sixty-five and over.

The second amendment established Medicaid, a Federal-state program to help provide medical services to the needy.

Medicare now covers 20 million elderly persons with tax-paid hospital benefits, plus optional insurance that can be purchased to help meet doctors' bills. Much of the opposition that greeted Medicare at the outset has dwindled.

Medicaid, on the other hand, has been criticized in several directions—for poor administrative procedures, for spending more on nursing homes than on physicians for the poor and for leaving low-income families vulnerable to heavy medical bills.

As costs of Medicare and Medicaid have rocketed to the fourteen-billion-dollar-a-year level, pressure has increased to revamp them and try to improve the efficiency of the programs.

Chief difficulty: Greater demands have been put on the already overburdened health system than it can meet.

Says Merle A. Gulick, vice president of the Equitable Life Assurance Society of the United States:

"It is . . . significant that all medical care prices have accelerated since 1966, the year Medicare began. Hospital prices have risen at the rate of about 15 per cent, and other medical care components have risen about 6 per cent."

"Exercise in Futility"

Jerome Pollack, associate dean of Harvard medical school, comments:

"The whole history of private insurance and of Medicare and Medicaid has been a cumulative exercise in the futility of acting solely on financing."

Dean Pollack and other medical authorities suggest that any broad health insurance program that does not also provide for expansion of all the nation's medical and hospital resources will be doomed to failure.

Among the needs these experts see:

> Physicians' aides with authority to perform relatively simple medical tasks, freeing doctors and nurses for more complicated work
>
> Wider use of group practice
>
> Greater reliance on outpatient clinics, with a stress on preventive health care
>
> Steps to broaden medical-education facilities
>
> Provision of more hospitals, nursing homes and the staffs to serve them

Whatever the outcome of the drive for a national health care system, one thing seems certain: The average man can expect his medical bills to go still higher in days to come.

A medical educator puts it this way:

"Advancing technology and rising demand for top-quality health care make it certain that costs are going to keep rising. That will be true whether the bills are paid in premiums for private insurance, or in taxes to support a public program."

WHAT ARE MEDICAID AND MEDICARE? [2]

Government, principally through Medicare and Medicaid, has ventured into paying some of the medical bills of those least able to pay—the elderly and the poor. Medicare includes two related programs for insuring persons over sixty-five against the costs of hospitalization, physicians' services and related health care. There is no means test. Part A, Hospital Insurance Benefits, covers practically all persons over age sixty-five. It draws its money from a special hospital insurance trust fund, in the case of Social Security beneficiaries, and general revenues, in the case of those not

[2] From "Paying More, Getting Less" (Part I of "The Growing Pains of Medical Care," a three-part article), by Fred Anderson, staff associate of the National Academy of Engineering. *New Republic.* 162:17-18. Ja. 17, '70. Reprinted by Permission of The New Republic, © 1970, Harrison-Blaine of New Jersey, Inc.

currently covered by Social Security. Part B, medical insurance for some (but nothing like all) physicians' fees and related costs, is financed by voluntary individual monthly payments, although the Federal Government also contributes from general revenues. Medicare functions quite smoothly, though hospitals complain of the paperwork and restrictions, and patients complain that in some hospitals they are discriminated against as Medicare patients. Lastly, and contrary to general belief, Medicare covers only about 35 per cent of the total health bill of persons over sixty-five.

Medicaid is more complicated. The primary recipients here are, in the bureaucratic phrase, the indigent "categorically needy": the aged, the blind, the disabled, and families with dependent children. Each participating state must submit a plan, and the categorically needy must be included. States are permitted, but not required, to include persons who are self-supporting but have no reserves to meet medical expenses. These are (again, their phrase) the "medically needy." States may also extend Medicaid to those whose only qualification is poverty. But the Federal Government will pay only the administrative costs of providing them with medical care. State Medicaid plans must offer five basic services: inpatient hospital care, outpatient hospital care, other lab and X-ray services, nursing-home services, and physicians' services. States may elect to provide five additional services for a comprehensive program.

WHAT'S WRONG WITH MEDICARE AND MEDICAID? [3]

These programs are criticized by medical economists because:

Like so many insurance programs and insurance-inspired projects, Medicare and Medicaid work more to protect the

[3] From *The Health of the Poor,* by Irvin Block, medical affairs writer. (Pamphlet no 435) Public Affairs Committee, Inc. 381 Park Ave. S. New York 10016. '69. p 18-19. Reprinted by permission.

one who provides the service than the one who gets the care. For many, these programs have meant no increase either in the quantity or the quality of medical services, only that the doctor or hospital clinic that formerly provided the service without charge would now get paid. While it is only right that medical practitioners should be paid for their services, this is not the overriding problem in the health of the poor. Seeing that doctors get paid their fees and improving the health of the poor are two different objectives.

In those cases where the availability of Medicare and Medicaid funds may have encouraged some poor to seek long-delayed medical attention that they would not have sought on their own, the result has been to place additional strain on the scarce manpower of the traditional sources of medical care. Back again to the problem that, given the old way of organizing medical care, there simply aren't enough doctors to go around.

Further, these programs do little or nothing about the accessibility, quality, or style of medical care delivered. They pay for services rendered by the piecemeal hospital clinics, by neighborhood loners who are often not competent to deal with complex diseases, and by doctors whose real skill and honesty do not make up for a lack of time, equipment, or organization to do a proper comprehensive job. Transportation costs are not reimbursed. Freedom to choose your own doctor is a slogan with a fine resonant ring, but it does not rate highest priority among poor people who have little experience of choosing or rating doctors and no understanding of what is truly meant by comprehensive care. How many people do? And it is comprehensive care—complete management and informed direction of a patient's health needs, in the context of his family and community—that is the next best step in improving medical care for the rich or the poor.

NATIONAL HEALTH CARE: HOW IT WORKS IN OTHER LANDS [4]

If the United States decides to relinquish its special status as the only major Western nation that has no state-assisted national health care plan for the great bulk of its citizens, it will be looking abroad at the ways in which others have handled the health care problem. And judging by what others have done, these are some of the lessons to be learned:

No fancy theoretical scheme can be imposed on a country. The plan must evolve from whatever health care structure is already there.

Every scheme that others have tried has serious imperfections. All are very difficult to manage.

Attempts to set up these schemes produce an enormous amount of bickering, but after a while both doctors and the public give it solid backing. London's Dr. M. R. Salkind, former secretary of Britain's General Practitioners' Association, sums it up: We must have national health. Private health is just too expensive."

The Canadian Scheme

Canada's national scheme may well be closest to any national plan that is likely to emerge in the United States. The Canadian scheme started operating on July 1, 1968, but it was designed to include the country's ten provincial governments. So far, 7 of the 10 have joined. The big breakthrough came last October 1 [1969] when Ontario finally signed up. It is Ontario that is most industrialized, most populous, and most like the United States.

In Ontario, a battle had raged over the role that private insurance companies would play in the scheme. The fighting ended in a peace pact between public and private

[4] From "The $60-Billion Crisis Over Medical Care." *Business Week*. p 54-5. Ja. 17, '70. Reprinted from the January 17, 1970 issue of *Business Week* by special permission. Copyrighted © 1970 by McGraw-Hill, Inc.

insurance interests. Under the pact, thirty-one private insurance companies were grouped in a nonprofit agency
called Healthco to act as administrators of the plan. Healthco handles the bulk of the paperwork in return for about
7 per cent of the premiums paid by Ontario's citizens.

Costs

In Canada, medical costs are lower than in the United
States. But they are comparable. Under the scheme, a family
that pays $14.75 a month is covered for doctor visits, sur-
gery, and various diagnostic and lab tests. For another $11.80
under a separate plan, the family gets coverage for hospital
ward costs, ambulance needs, physiotherapy, and other care.
The companies in Healthco are still free to sell insurance
for items not covered by the basic plan, and the market
is strong.

The Canadian scheme rests primarily on the provincial
governments. But an average of 50 per cent of the cost will
be paid by the federal government—more for the poorer
provinces, less for the richer ones. To participate, each
province's health plan must cover at least 90 per cent of its
population, include a wide range of services, and be run by
a nonprofit agency.

Ontario's Health Department reports that, since October
1, it has been paying out more than $1 million in claims
daily. It estimates total claims for the first year will be about
$415 million. With administrative and other expenses, total
outlays should be $508 million. To finance the plan, Ontario
will get $168 million from Ottawa, $309 million in premiums, and the balance from its own government.

The scheme pays doctors 90 per cent of their fees, which
are set by their own medical association. Under old pri-
vate-insurance schemes, the 90 per cent rule had always
held good. But now that the entire population is involved,
trade unions and other groups are agitating for 100 per
cent payment. Meanwhile, doctors try to collect the unpaid

10 per cent from patients, generating some confusion and ill will.

The British Plan

In Britain, the National Health Service also generates wrangling among doctors, patients, and health authorities. But the trouble dates back before 1948, the year the health service was set up. Long before that, British medicine had split into three different establishments:

> General practitioners, who perform 90 per cent of all medical care but are barred from treating their patients in hospitals
>
> Hospitals, now old and rundown, which are staffed by high-paid specialists, low-paid juniors, and badly paid nurses
>
> Local health authorities, county and municipal groups, which run clinics, child welfare, and ambulance services

British GPs work basically for salaries paid by the health service. Only 20 per cent of them earn income from private practice, too. Eight years ago, thousands of them protested bitterly over their salary levels and threatened to resign from the health service. But since then the rates have been changed. GPs now rank fifth among British salaried professionals, though their salaries are still low by U.S. doctors' standards.

The bitterest rift over pay is in British hospitals. There, specialists who win consulting posts can pull in up to $25,000 a year, plus extra money from private practice. But there is a limit of 10,000 on the number of specialists who may be employed in the hospitals. Other doctors, just as fully qualified, may wait half their working lives for a consultant's spot to open up while drawing a top salary of just $6,900 a year.

About six hundred British doctors emigrate every year, many of them simply because of frustration over pay. And only about two thousand new doctors graduate from British

medical schools each year. Supply and demand would hav‹
gotten hopelessly out of whack years ago, and the Nationa
Health Service would probably have broken down, wer‹
it not for the two-thousand-odd doctors who migrate t‹
Britain each year, mostly from Commonwealth nations.

Even so, one of the hallmarks of the service is constan
delay. For health service patients, the waiting time fo:
minor surgery can run to months, even to a year and more

This is where private health insurance goes to work i1
Britain. A private patient who is ready to pay is assigne‹
to a different waiting list. He gets one of a fixed number o‹
hospital beds set aside for paying patients. Or he may choos‹
to enter a privately owned clinic.

So, company-paid health insurance is now the mark o
executive status in Britain. Some nine thousand companie:
buy these policies to make sure that their hospitalized execu
tives get immediate admission, private rooms, telephones
and TV sets. About 2 million Britons hold private policie
today compared with just 86,000 when the national systen
was set up in 1948.

The largest health insurance company in Britain i:
the British United Provident Association, whose 1969 in
come was some $36 million, mostly from group coverage
A typical family premium is $105 a year.

Sweden

When Sweden set up its national health plan in 1955
it did not encounter the condemnation by doctors that the
British and Canadian plans met when they were started
Some 70 per cent of Swedes were already in various volun
tary health insurance schemes and, for doctors, the change
largely meant switching from one set of forms to another.

But Sweden's plan, too, has run into problems. There
are long waiting lists for surgery, long lineups at clinics,
complaints of impersonal treatment at big-city hospitals.

At the root of the Swedish troubles is a worldwide prob-

em: the shortage of medical staff. In some Swedish prov-
nces, hospitals have to close in the summer for staff vaca-
ions.

Paperwork is the second bane of the Swedish system.
3ut the government may have an answer. Starting July 1
1970], each patient will pay a fee of $1.50 to $2 each time
e makes a routine visit to a doctor, hospital, or clinic.
'ew administrative papers will be filled out for such visits,
nd the saving in red tape should make the whole system
ess costly.

THE CASE FOR NATIONAL HEALTH INSURANCE [5]

Foreign observers visiting the United States to examine
he method of payment for medical services would find it
lifficult to conduct their inquiry. They would discover that
n health, as in a variety of other fields, answers they receive
o questions would depend on where and of whom the
questions were asked. Some individuals pay or purchase in-
urance for medical care out of their own incomes. Various
evels of government pay for some kinds of care for some
people. Private charity provides certain services to certain
groups. Not only do different sources pay for medical expenses for different persons, but multiple sources often pay
for different parts of the care for an individual and family.
Eligibility for payment by the various systems depends on
the person's age, income, health condition, and on standards
set by different levels of government, place of residence, and
sundry other variables.

Only a discreet and diplomatic observer would say the
situation is confused. A less tactful person might simply
say, "It is a mess." He would be correct.

In general, the medical care delivery and payment system is based on a philosophy that medical care is a private

[5] From article by Rashi Fein, professor of the economics of medicine, Harvard University. Saturday Review. 53:27-9+. Ag. 22, '70. Copyright 1970 Saturday Review, Inc. Reprinted by permission.

matter: Providers of care have the right to select the in
dividuals to whom they render care, and the consumer ha
the responsibility to pay for the care he seeks. Govern
ment is only a "court of last resort." It intervenes when hel
is sorely needed and, generally, only when the normal mar
ket has demonstrated its inadequacy. In recent years, sucl
help has become increasingly necessary, as evidenced b
two major medical care financing programs: Medicare an
Medicaid. Yet, even Medicare and Medicaid can hardl
be considered adequate to meet the payment needs of th
population they serve, let alone of all those who need help

In earlier years, there were many who felt that the pay
ment-for-services problem could be solved by voluntar
health insurance. They drew an analogy to fire or thef
insurance, which protects the individual against a high
cost catastrophe with a very low probability of occurrence
Thus, if all individuals contributed small amounts, protec
tion would be available for the few who were hit by a
disaster not of their own making. Health insurance, how
ever, turned out to be different. The probabilities were no
so low (and for, say, physicians' visits, were quite high)
some events against which protection was sought did no
have catastrophic monetary consequences (again physicians'
visits, for example); and utilization of services and there
fore of coverage was controlled to some extent by the in
dividual and to a large extent by the provider, making the
probabilities in part dependent on whether the individual
had coverage. Consequently, voluntary health insurance
came to look more and more like a budgeting system for
health expenditures rather than insurance.

The problem of financing insurance coverage is becoming more severe. Although family income in the United
States has been rising, medical care prices have been increasing even more rapidly, and more and more families
are finding it difficult to pay for insurance. Further, many
individuals who need financial protection are viewed as
"uninsurable," since their medical conditions make high

xpenditures predictable. Inclusion of "high-risk" persons
with other subscribers means higher premiums; excluding
hem leaves those who are most vulnerable to fend for them-
elves.

The aged, for example, use many more health services
han does the younger population. Therefore, commercial
nsurers developed premium structures for population
groups that did not include the aged. This, in turn, led to
a siphoning-off of persons likely to have the most favorable
experience, and left those with likely unfavorable experience
n a weak position. Blue Cross programs that had begun
with "community rating" (everyone in a community paid
he same rate) lost subscribers who could obtain lower
rates from carriers that did not cover the old. As a higher
and higher proportion of Blue Cross subscribers became
persons likely to have an unfavorable experience, premiums
rose. In the absence of a social insurance philosophy that
requires compulsory coverage, this situation creates havoc.

The remaining difficulty with voluntary private insurance
is that, as structured, it offers little incentive toward economy and efficiency in provision of health services, or toward substitution of less expensive services for more expensive ones. In medical care, a field controlled by professionals and one in which the consumer often lacks knowledge, private health insurers have tended to be nothing
more than bill payers. They have watched prices rise, but
have done little to exert leverage on behalf of subscribers.
Furthermore, insurance has provided built-in incentives for
use of high-cost hospital services rather than ambulatory
services. Given the traditions of the voluntary private health
insurance sector, it is doubtful that it could be a force toward rationalization of the health care system. Voluntary
private insurance cannot be considered as the vehicle for
financing medical care for the American people. . . .

Opposition to national health insurance will come from
various sources. Some will suggest that, whatever its future

merits, the nation is not yet prepared for it; that we mus
get ready for the increase in demand the program woul
bring; that we must first increase the supply of personne
and facilities and rationalize and reorganize the system t
achieve greater productivity. I submit that if we choose t
wait till we are better prepared, we will wait a very lon
time. What, after all, has the Administration done, wha
is it proposing to do, to increase resources and rationaliz
the system during the "waiting period"? Little will happe
to improve the situation, and we shall find ourselves n
more ready for national health insurance six years fror
now than we are today.

There is little evidence to suggest that, as a nation, w
do well in "getting ready" for the future. If we respond a
all, we do so when the problem is upon us. We commit re
sources to increasing supply only when the demand has a
ready been there; when the public has been frustrated i
its ability to find services that have been promised. We mus
mobilize demand if we want to bring changes in supply

Finally—and this lies at the center of the debate—to sa
that we are not yet ready to institute a national healt
program is to say that even today we cannot deliver th
medical care that Americans need. If that is the case, i
the system is unable to produce more services, shall w
continue to ration the short supply on the basis of incom
and ability to pay for the services? Is this the basis on which
medical care should be distributed? Should we not ratio
according to medical need?

I believe that we should commit ourselves to the con
cept of a national health insurance program and mov
forward to institute it as rapidly as it can be enacted. W
must begin the debate. The submission of specific legis
lative proposals helps to focus the debate. Important as i
is to enact national health insurance as rapidly as possible
it is also important that we not enter the political-bar

;aining stage before we examine the issues. It is important
hat all of us increase our understanding of the advantages
ind disadvantages of various options. Only in this way will
ve who are not part of the legislative process or members
»f organizations with links to the process make an impact
»n the design of an equitable program that protects against
he financial burden of high medical costs and promotes de-
elopment of a health care system that meets the needs of
»ur population.

THE CASE AGAINST NATIONAL HEALTH INSURANCE [6]

The hottest topic in medical legislation today is the
:reeping plague of socialized medicine. Its most recent dis-
;uise is in the form of a national health insurance program
or everyone, sometimes in conjunction with a prepaid
iealth care plan. One program that would completely re-
«tructure the present delivery of health care is the one
:ntitled "Health Security Program" recently introduced by
senator [Edward M.] Kennedy [Democrat, Massachusetts]
ind Congresswoman Martha [W.] Griffith [Democrat, Michi-
;an], which is the Reuther Plan and is backed by AFL-CIO.
The common cry of all of these programs is "Better Health
Care at Lower Cost." This is a laudable goal, and everyone
should work toward it, but let's see where we're going
»efore we jump off the cliff. The [California Professional]
Guild has made an in-depth study of the subject and some
of the flaws in the various programs being advanced are so
obvious that it is hard to believe they are not being pre-
ented with tongue-in-cheek. Let's examine a few of the main
weaknesses. First, who are the masterminds who are planning the future of American medicine?

[6] From "The Health Security Program," speech delivered by Paul Ashton,
M.D., president of the California Professional Guild, before the California Pro-
essional Guild at Newport Beach, California, September 9, 1970. *Vital Speeches
of the Day*. 37:100-2. D. 1, 70. Reprinted by permission.

A new breed of experts has arrived on the scene. A highly educated group of technocrats, system analysts, economists statisticians, social planners and administrators—a new race of healthocrats—and they are going to solve the nation' health care problems because they have had special course and studies to equip them for this monumental task? These self-appointed guardians of our nation's health boldly say that *we* (the medical profession) are too simple-minded to be entrusted with such a mission; consequently, there isn' a fumbling physician, a feeble pharmacist or a doddering dentist in the bunch. We have the experience, but they are going to save the world for us—and from us. The writing is on the wall, big and bold: "They (meaning all medical men) will no longer have a voice in the shape of the systems under which they practice." Here are a few direct quotes:

The institutions and organizations of the medical community must respond to the challenges of the times. If they refuse, their punishment will be to live under the judgment of less knowledgeable men than themselves. Indifference to the social issues of medicine will ultimately guarantee government intervention . . . this is not a threat, but a realistic assessment of current trends. (John G. Veneman, Undersecretary of HEW, former California Assemblyman)

We are coming to recognize that there has to be a great deal more in-depth planning for the distribution of health care and manpower, and that this doesn't necessarily require medical knowledge. (HEW Deputy Undersecretary Frederic V. Malek, former toolmaker)

I cannot help feeling that a major reason doctors have not had greater influence on such matters is that they have usually not had enough educational background in the economic and social aspects of medical care to be able to grapple with this kind of issue. . . . If the physician wants to be one of the molders of policy he is going to have to be equipped to do so. (Rashi Fein of the Harvard Center for Community Health and Medical Care)

The Healthocrats say they advocate "no formal Federal takeover of hospitals, no socialization of doctors . . . nor any compulsion." *Who's kidding whom?*

Let's examine the first part of the slogan—"Better Health Care at Lower Cost." It is impossible to provide medical are to everyone in the country because there are simply not nough primary physicians to go around? If our medical chools would turn out more primary physicians, the natural aw of competition fostered under the free enterprise system vould take care of better physician distribution and better are to outlying areas. But until the experts realize this laring deficiency in their planning, their program will just ave to work with what doctors we now have.

Statistics from other countries show the patient load ncreases dramatically under socialized medical plans. Why an't we learn from this? In other countries, including some f the Canadian provinces that have similar health insurnce programs, it has been shown that the patient load has ncreased tenfold; yet, interestingly enough, there has been o corresponding increase in the number of hospitalizations. This would indicate that there are no more really "sick" eople—just more patients.

It's human nature for people to want something "free" vhether they need it or not. So, if you are seeing around 40 atients a day now, you will be expected to see around 400 nder the national health insurance program. And babies ith diarrhea may have to wait weeks for an appointment ecause you are too busy with patients who need their Band-Aids changed. How can we handle such a patient load nd call it "better care"? You will have to go into your aiting room and say, "All right, everyone with a backche please stand up." Then you can give some group iagnosis and distribute printed sheets of do's and don'ts or back problems. Of course, if the program has enough oney in it for X rays, then everyone in the group will et them—whether or not they are indicated. And there ill be no time to help those who suffer from fear, loneness, guilt, anxiety, or any other "illness" that is not on e fee schedule. And what about Grandma Jones who needs er gall bladder removed but your budget is overdrawn or the year—will she have her cholecystectomy or will the operations be postponed until the next fiscal year when the new funds are appropriated? . . .

When any system prevents the personal one-to-one relationship between patient and doctor, with continuity of that care by the same doctor, then it is less than the best. Nothing will ever replace the doctor sitting down with a patient in an examining room and listening to his history, complaints and problems. And it must be the same doctor with the same patient, year after year—one who knows his personality, his family, his history, his peculiar foibles and anxieties. To change this personal relationship for assembly line care would be disastrous. The only conclusion is that patient care will *not* be improved—it will deteriorate. Now what about the claim of lower costs?

A vast new bureaucracy will administer health care to over 200 million people with all the present Medicare services, plus preventive medicine, plus predictive medicine, plus many other benefits and it will be for everyone, regardless of age or income, with no exclusions or deductions. This is the great giveaway . . . the biggest bargain since Barnum and Bailey. Again, we say: *"Who is kidding whom?"* Who is going to pay for the health clinics that must be built (about two thousand of them planned across the country, many of them duplicating present facilities)? Who is going to pay for the organization costs . . . the high salaries of the Healthocrats . . . the administrative costs . . . the crushing load of paper work? The employers are supposed to pay 35 per cent of the bill through a payroll tax, the employees will pay 25 per cent of the costs, and the Government is supposed to pay the remaining 40 per cent. Of course, this 40 per cent will be passed on to the public, making double payments by the taxpayers. Sounds like an automobile pitch! The demonstration ride is free, but who is going to make the monthly payments?

Last year [1969] $67 billion were paid to the health industry by everyone, including the Government, private citizens and insurance companies. This is big business. Now the figures being tossed into the health hopper are that the budget will be only $37 billion—a *savings* of $30 billion—yet everything will be *free* to everyone. And all this will be accomplished by the magic of a medical budget. We recognize and agree with the crying need to provide medical care to the underprivileged and the poor, but the planning outlined by these social engineers will only compound the problems, and we resent the silly games they are playing with such vital issues. They cry "economics," but it makes one wonder if it isn't more political than economical? Is their goal really health to the poor, or votes at the polls? Could it also be a tool to demand the loyalty of the blue-collar worker? And even if their program was economically sound, how would it be administered?

The Healthocrats are going to show us how to do it. [For a presentation of proposed organization and of the basic philosophy behind the original idea here objected to, see "The Patient as a Consumer," below, in Section IV.—Ed.] They say there will be no formal takeover and no compulsion, but what do you call it when all policies and administration is set by the Government? You will be handed a prepackaged program and will submit annual budgets for health care to be reviewed by the Healthocrats. If your costs run over your budget, then you just fill in form No. 988654709962F-aS, and in about three years you might get partial payment. *You conform or you don't get paid.* It's that simple. And these trained brains say the Government can streamline health care delivery into an efficient operation. Do you agree? Federal expertise in "health care" has already been proven —just look at the Veterans Hospitals. And as for their experience in "delivery," well, the Government operates a unique *mail* delivery, so why wouldn't they do as well with *health care* delivery. Put the two departments together and we will have a sort of *Medical Post Office.*

THE CASE FOR A NATIONAL HEALTH
INSURANCE PARTNERSHIP [7]

In recent years, a new method for delivering health services has achieved growing respect. This new approach has two essential attributes. It brings together a comprehensive range of medical services in a single organization so that a patient is assured of convenient access to all of them. And it provides needed services for a fixed contract fee which is paid in advance by all subscribers.

Such an organization can have a variety of forms and names and sponsors. One of the strengths of this new concept, in fact, is its great flexibility. The general term which has been applied to all of these units is "HMO"—Health Maintenance Organization.

Under traditional systems, doctors and hospitals are paid in effect, on a piecework basis. The more illnesses they treat, and the more service they render, the more their income rises. This does not mean, of course, that they do any less than their very best to make people well. But it does mean that there is no economic incentive for them to concentrate on keeping people healthy.

A fixed-price contract for comprehensive care reverses this illogical incentive. Under this arrangement, income grows not with the number of days a person is sick but with the number of days he is well.

Patients and practitioners alike are enthusiastic about this organizational concept. So is this Administration. That is why we proposed legislation . . . [in] March [1970] to enable Medicare recipients to join such programs. That is why I am now making the following additional recommendations:

We should require public and private health insurance plans to allow beneficiaries to use their plan to purchase

[7] From President Richard M. Nixon's message to Congress, February 18, 1971, urging "a new national health strategy." Text from the New York *Times.* p 16. F. 19, '71.

membership in a Health Maintenance Organization when one is available.

To help new HMOs get started—an expensive and complicated task—we should establish a new $23 million program of planning grants to aid potential sponsors in both the private and public sector.

We should provide additional support to help sponsors raise the necessary capital, construct needed facilities and sustain initial operating deficits until they achieve an enrollment which allows them to pay their own way. . . .

In the last twenty years, the segment of our population owning health insurance has grown from 50 per cent to 87 per cent and the portion of medical bills paid for by insurance has gone from 35 per cent to 60 per cent. But despite this impressive growth, there are still serious gaps in present health insurance coverage.

I am proposing that a National Health Insurance Standards Act be adopted which will require employers to provide basic health insurance coverage for their employees.

In the past, we have taken similar actions to assure workers a minimum wage, to provide them with disability and retirement benefits and to set occupational health and safety standards. Now we should go one step further and guarantee that all workers will receive adequate health insurance protection.

I am also proposing that a new family health insurance plan be established to meet the special needs of poor families, who would not be covered by the proposed National Health Insurance Standards Act, headed by unemployed or self-employed persons.

The Medicaid program was designed to help these people, but—for many reasons—it has not accomplished its goals.

Our program would also require the establishment in each state of special insurance pools which would offer insurance at reasonable group rates to people who did not qualify for other programs: the self-employed, for example and poor-risk individuals who often cannot get insurance

I also urge the Congress to take further steps to im prove Medicare. For one thing, beneficiaries should be allowed to use the program to join Health Maintenance Organizations. In addition, we should consolidate the finan cing of Part A of Medicare—which pays for hospital care —and Part B—which pays for outpatient services, provided the elderly person himself pays a monthly fee to qualify for this protection. . . .

Nineteen months ago I said that America's medical sys stem faced a massive crisis. Since that statement was made that crisis has deepened. All of us must now join together in a common effort to meet this crisis—each doing his own part to mobilize more effectively the enormous potential of our health care system.

HEALTH CARE WITHOUT MIRACLES [8]

Our present system of medical care is not a system at all. The majority of physicians, operating alone as private entrepreneurs, constitute an army of pushcart vendors in an age of supermarkets. Most patients pay by the cumber some fee-for-service or piecework method, which involve separate billing for visits to doctors, shots, X rays, labora tory tests, surgery, anesthesia, hospital room and board etc., etc. The American hospital system, as Herman M. and Anne R. Somers of Princeton University said in their book *Medicare and the Hospitals,* "is largely a figure of speech," the result of a haphazard growth of isolated, uncoordinated institutions. . . .

Even when doctors have the best of motives, as a ma jority of them doubtless do, this lax competitive climat discourages the efficiency that comes with cost-consciou

[8] From article "Better Care at Less Cost Without Miracles," by Edmun K. Faltermayer, member of *Fortune* Board of Editors. *Fortune.* 81:80-3+. Ja '70. Courtesy of Fortune Magazine.

ıess. And even if the doctor has a conscience about wasting he money of patient, government, or insurance company, he growing menace of malpractice suits may induce him o pile on precautionary tests and treatments—which he an do without restraint. "Almost nowhere else in the ːconomy," says Victor R. Fuchs, a leading economist at he National Bureau of Economic Research, "do tech- ıologists have as much control over demand." The only ˈarallel, Fuchs says, is the military's control of the de- ˈense budget in time of total war.

The growth of "third party" payment of medical bills hrough Blue Cross, Blue Shield, and group insurance ˈolicies has provided another inflationary thrust. Until ˈery recently the Blues and the insurance companies, ˈvhich now disburse about $13 billion a year, have directed ˈery little hard scrutiny at fees or the quantity of the ˈervices that they are buying. They have contented them- ˈelves instead with the role of a largely automatic "cost- ˈass-through" mechanism. In the past, some check on ˈosts came from individual patients complaining about ˈiigh bills. Doctors and hospitals had to worry about the ˈinancial hardship that the larding on of services might ˈreate. But the emergence of large, "rich," impersonal in- ˈurers has removed even these controls. . . .

Henry J.'s New Model

Those patterns, however, are not like the laws of the Medes and the Persians—they need not stand forever. Evidence that they can be changed, with benefits for all the parties involved—doctors, patients, and insurers—is piling up. Some eight million Americans now receive medical care under plans that work well, and that are subject to the constraints of the marketplace. These "pre- paid group-practice" plans are not the only model for re- form. Further, even these plans have not yet been brought to the degree of efficiency that they may someday reach.

Nevertheless, they represent an alternative that more Ameri
cans should be able to choose. Their expansion woulc
exert a badly needed competitive discipline upon the res
of the medical system.

The Kaiser Foundation program is by far the larges
of the prepaid systems. It has two million members an
its own network of hospitals and outpatient clinics in Ca
ifornia, Oregon, and Hawaii. The program began in th
late 1930s when the late Henry J. Kaiser, then buildin
hydroelectric dams in remote locations, felt obliged t
provide medical services for construction workers and thei
families. After a conventional, fee-for-service payment sy
tem proved unpopular, Kaiser substituted a single fee cover
ing all needed services, and the plan was enthusiasticall
accepted. In response to requests from hundreds of forme
shipyard workers, Kaiser kept the program going on th
West Coast after 1945, and opened it to the general public
Today, employees of the various Kaiser companies and thei
families constitute only about 3 per cent of the membership

The Kaiser plan has made some notable improvement
over the orthodox means of distributing medical care. T
begin with, access is easy. Physicians of all major specialtie
are housed in large clinics in each of the regions covere
by the plan. A middle-aged man with an abdominal pai
can see his internist and can be referred within minute
to another specialist in the same building, which has it
own X ray and laboratories. If the patient requires ho
pitalization, he is sent to one of the Kaiser Foundation'
nineteen hospitals, many of which adjoin the outpatien
clinics.

Unlike ordinary private "health insurance," which i
really sickness insurance designed to reimburse selecte
medical expenses under the fee-for-service system, th
Kaiser program assumes broad responsibility for keepin
its members sound of body. The range of services varie
according to the employer group or individual membe

ut a fairly typical plan offered in the San Francisco-Sacamento area currently costs a total of $35.40 a month or a subscriber with two or more dependents, including he employer's contribution. This covers all professional ervices in the hospital, in the doctor's office, and in the ome, including surgery; all X-ray and laboratory services; ll preventive care, including physical examinations; and ospital care for up to 111 days per person in a calendar ear. Some nominal charges are made for drugs and for octors' visits ($1 per office visit, and up to $5 for house alls after 5:00 P.M.), and there is a $60 charge for maternity care. Some items are excluded, notably dental care, sychiatry, and nursing-home care (though some Kaiser lans offer psychiatric and convalescent care, too). For an dditional monthly payment of 15 cents, hospitalization can e extended all the way to 365 days.

A Reward for Cutting Costs

The more liberal of the Kaiser plans probably cover bout three quarters of a family's insurable medical expenses. The very breadth of the coverage provides two mportant benefits. On the one hand, no paid-up member eed be deterred from seeking medical care for fear of the xpense. On the other hand, no built-in bias exists favoring a particular *type* of care, since most types are covered nyway. A patient does not have to be admitted to a hosital for a test or a minor operation, which could be given n an ambulatory basis, solely in order to gain insurance overage.

The Kaiser plan also provides an incentive for efficiency. he providers of medical care—the doctors and the hositals—*share* the financial risks of illness with the patient. Members' monthly charges are set for a year, and during at period the program must operate on the revenue enerated by these charges. If costs exceed revenues during at period, the Kaiser system must absorb them. . . .

Practicing "Pure Medicine"

Kaiser's experience refutes the widely held belief that if medical services are "free," or virtually free, the public will stampede to them. Neither does the evidence indicate that Kaiser has gone to the opposite extreme, cutting corners and denying needed medical care. This criticism is often voiced by doctors opposed to prepaid group practice along with the familiar charge that group practice precludes the free choice of "family" physician, and that it renders care in an impersonal, "assembly-line" manner which lowers the quality of medical services.

In fact, the Kaiser program makes possible an educated choice of a family physician, because the patient in a large clinic is in a position to compare doctors. The atmosphere at one Kaiser clinic, in suburban Walnut Creek, California, is a good deal less suggestive of an assembly line than the typical jammed office of a solo practitioner; the place has more the relaxed ambience of a resort inn. . . . One factor raising quality, according to Dr. Wallace H. Cook, the suntanned physician in chief of the Walnut Creek Center, is that doctors devote themselves to "absolutely pure medicine here." They have nothing to do with the billing and they do not have to worry about the financial impact of the type of care that they prescribe on the patient, since virtually all phases of medical care are prepaid. . . .

Another advantage that Kaiser physicians enjoy over their counterparts in solo practice is access to good health records. Generally, health records are in a medieval state, with incomplete data on each individual scattered in every doctor's office and hospital that he has ever visited. Most Kaiser members' medical histories are readily retrievable and in a growing number of cases are stored on computer tapes. The eventual goal is to give each member a lifetime electronic medical file, based in part on the periodic multiphasic testing with which the Kaiser Foundation is now experimenting on a large scale.

Probably the greatest spur to maintaining the quality of medical services is the fact that Kaiser does not have a monopoly over health care in the areas it serves. Once a year each group, and each individual within a group, has the chance to drop out of the program if he wishes. If enrollment figures are any guide, the consumers couldn't be happier. Membership has grown threefold in the last ten years, and the Kaiser Foundation is expanding about as fast as its financial resources will permit, currently at a rate of 200,000 persons a year. It has recently moved east of the Rockies to start a health plan in Denver, and to team up with a group plan in Cleveland. . . .

While some of the other group plans have matched or even exceeded Kaiser's cost savings, they have not enjoyed the same rapid growth in membership. Detroit's Community Health Association, whose rolls have been static for several years, is hampered in part by its "union" label that deters white-collar and other middle-class workers from joining. New York's HIP [Health Insurance Plan] has been stalled at approximately its present membership for the past year or so, and some unions have withdrawn from the plan. HIP has been handicapped because until recently it did not own its own hospitals; it simply referred patients to community hospitals and paid the bill. In some cases its doctors handled HIP members along with nonmembers paying on a fee-for-service basis. As a result, HIP members have often been kept waiting, and some of them, says a spokesman for a union that recently pulled out, "felt they were being treated as second-class citizens."

Elsewhere around the country, new group-practice programs are getting under way. The main impetus is coming from teaching hospitals—which until now have remained aloof from the nitty-gritty of community health services—and some of the insurance carriers. The new Harvard Community Health Plan, which hopes to attract members from the entire Boston area, is the outgrowth of years of soul searching by the Harvard Medical School on the mission of the medical school and the hospital. Jerome Pollack, associate dean of Harvard Medical School who designed the new program, has combined some existing institutions—four community hospitals that will accept patients from the new program—with a newly opened outpatient clinic operated by the plan itself and staffed mainly with salaried physicians. With premiums set at $50 a month per family irrespective of size, the coverage will be somewhat broader than Kaiser's: patients will be eligible for fairly extensive psychiatric care, as well as convalescent care in nursing homes.

Pollack expects the plan to break even in about three years, by which time he hopes enrollment will have reached 30,000. Instead of bypassing the insurance companies, as the Kaiser program does, Pollack has enlisted their help in canvasing members from among those already signed up under existing programs. Blue Cross is expected to supply 70 per cent of the members and a group of ten commercial insurance companies—including such giants in the health field as Aetna, Metropolitan, Equitable, and Travelers— will supply the rest. Pollack is aiming for a cross section of all income groups and races, in order to gain operating experience meaningful for the whole U.S. population. "We envision," he says, "something that the giant insurance companies and Blue Cross will be able to duplicate on a large scale."

The insurance companies have been initiating some experiments of their own. As President Charles A. Siegfried of Metropolitan Life concedes, the big carriers have until recently been "standoffish" about improving the nation's medical system. For a long time, he says, there was "a fatalistic acceptance of rising costs," and "we felt we shouldn't tell doctors how to run their services." All this is beginning to change. Following a meeting in Boston last October [1969], the Health Insurance Association of America, representing most of the commercial carriers, recommended that the companies "exert their influence to bring about soundly conceived changes" in the U.S. health system.

Metropolitan has already supplied funds for a new ambulatory care center at Washington University Medical School in St. Louis which will include a "demonstration" group-practice program. Equitable is providing most of the mortgage money for the construction of a combined neighborhood health center and nursing home that will house a new group-practice system in a Washington, D.C., Negro neighborhood. Perhaps the most deeply involved insurance company is Connecticut General, which is putting up $3.75 million of mortgage money for a clinic and hospital at the new town of Columbia, Maryland, which will serve members of a new prepaid group-practice plan. Connecticut General, which is also providing $500,000 of development costs, will have first crack at selling the plan, but its involvement stops short of actually setting it up and running it; Johns Hopkins Medical School in Baltimore will do that.

IV. HEALTH CARE AND THE COMMUNITY

EDITOR'S INTRODUCTION

In the past few years the public has increasingly made its voice heard in matters that have long been considered the exclusive concern of the doctor. No doubt even without this public pressure, changes in the delivery of medical care would have come about, for within the medical community itself new forces are stirring. Many concerned doctors and medical students are aware today as never before of social issues, largely because they have come to the belief that the social environment their patients live in has a direct and immediate effect on the quality of health care. Furthermore, the increasing interest of the community in its health care is a new factor and one of the major reasons why many observers believe that U.S. medicine now stands at the threshold of a period of revolutionary changes in its relationship with the community.

One product of this ferment has been the gradual acceptance of the concept of the citizen as a participant in the planning of health care. This is most clearly seen in community health centers which bring together under one roof medical professionals and specially trained nonprofessional aides, called paraprofessional or paramedical aides, from the community. Under this arrangement the community itself is not just a passive receiver of services. It takes an active role in health services, providing the paraprofessionals who do certain important and time-consuming tasks and thus enabling the doctor to devote undivided attention to medical tasks. Through its representatives, the community also has a voice in the center's operations, an arrangement which may prove a mixed blessing, as conflict between the medical professionals and the community paraprofessionals and executive staff will no doubt occur. Still, there may be some wider application for the community health centers beyond the urban slums where they are today sprouting up.

This fourth section is about some of the revolutionary changes underway in the traditional relationship between the medical practitioner and the community in which he practices. The first selection is an excerpt from the Report of the Task Force on Medicaid and Related Programs of the United States Department of Health, Education, and Welfare. It puts forward the somewhat surprising concept that a patient is not simply a patient. He is also a consumer of health services and as such is entitled to some of the protections to which most other consumers are entitled. Next, a selection excerpted from the *Carnegie Quarterly* discusses some of the problems of communication, both in language and in concept, between a middle-class doctor practicing in a slum and his patients. In the third article, Jeanne Bockel of *Science News* describes the recent growth of community medicine. Finally, medical writer Irvin Block describes some of the procedures and problems of organizing health care in the slums.

THE PATIENT AS A CONSUMER [1]

While the concept of citizen participation in the planning and policy-making processes of health institutions is not new, it has been limited largely to the professional, business, social, and other so-called leaders in a community with the users or other consumers excluded. The growing dissatisfaction with health care systems and the increasing demand for participation in the decision-making process is coming from many sources, but the newest voices are from low-income and minority groups, who until now have been largely passive recipients of health services. Recognizing the importance of

[1] From the *Report of the Task Force on Medicaid and Related Programs* [United States. Department of Health, Education, and Welfare]. Supt. of Docs. Washington, D.C. 20402. '70. p 71-3, 112-14.

these voices, recent legislation has emphasized a more force
ful role for consumers in determining how goals and policie
are set, how resources are allocated and programs and serv
ices operated.

The Task Force believes that one cause of the inade
quacies and dysfunctions in health services has been tha
those providing services have controlled the decision-making
process. Self-serving is sometimes the result, but there are
other possible consequences too, such as isolation from
knowledge about the medical and health needs of a pop
ulation.

Health professional workers have been reluctant to share
decision making in health policy and continue to regard
policy making as their traditional domain. Their reluctance
is based on the belief that consumers have insufficient knowl
edge to participate in decision making and are often unac
customed to the demands of institutionalized efforts.

There is some concern among providers that consumer
participation can delay decision making, and even a feeling
that a product of consumer participation may be dilution of
the quality of health care services. There is no nationa
means of providing the consumer the assistance he needs to
become a positive force for improving the nation's health
care services, nor does the means now exist for bringing the
consumer and provider together to work jointly for improve
ments.

One of the basic assumptions underlying this report i
that the consumer, defined as any user of the health care sys
tem, can be a responsible partner in a system that require
intelligent and caring people to make it work. The recom
mendations that follow assume that the consumer can help
to identify problems and inadequacies in medical care, car
suggest solutions and can help to design and implement new
policy.

To bring the consumer into the policy-making proces
will require: (a) strengthening existing consumer groups ir

health, welfare and related areas; (b) encouraging the establishment of new groups that are truly representative of the consumer point of view; and (c) developing formal working relationships between consumers and those responsible for the delivery and quality of health care.

Any board or group set up to advise policy-making officials at any level of government must provide for consumer representation to protect and present the interests and needs of the consumer. In addition, executive committees, subcommittees, and ad hoc committees of such boards or groups should have a significant number of consumer representatives as members.

The consumer members selected to serve on policy-making and advisory boards should reflect the social, economic, racial and geographic characteristics of their communities. They may be selected by their local constituencies, or from labor unions, consumer-sponsored, group-practice plans, or welfare-recipient organizations. Individuals directly involved in the provision, delivery, or administration of health care services should not be eligible to serve as consumer representatives unless they have been duly selected by *bona fide* consumer organizations which are aware of their involvement in health care delivery.

Any federally funded and/or operated health programs must provide for consumer participants on advisory committees and councils concerned with planning, purchasing and delivering health services.

Organizations and institutions involved in planning, purchasing, and delivering health services should provide for majority consumer participation in deliberations on the nature of those services, and at least one third of that majority should be made up of users of the health care program or facility involved. The provision of majority representation in which at least one third is composed of actual users should be a requirement for all organizations and institutions, but especially for those seeking Federal support for health care programs.

Proprietary organizations and institutions concerned with health care services, although not necessarily subject to regulations applying to grants and other support, should be encouraged to provide for consumer involvement in the monitoring of their services.

State agencies should be required by the Federal Government to have majority representation of consumers and consumer representatives on state advisory committees on Medicaid. . . .

Not only do millions of consumers get care on a hit-or-miss basis or lack access to care except in medical crises, but virtually all consumers lack access to the decision-making machinery that can bring about change. Few institutions and programs include representatives of everyday users of their services on policy-making or governing boards, in spite of their nonprofit and presumably "community" character.

The result is that medical care is still too often delivered at the time and place, and in the way convenient to provider rather than consumer. Old patterns persist in the face of new demands—a basic cause of rising dissatisfaction with the health services.

A basic tenet of the report is that greater consumer involvement in decision making is required to overcome deficiencies in the health system with reasonable dispatch and to achieve better management of resources. Without substantial consumer input, health institutions can become excessively self-serving and in fact, tangential to even fundamental community health problems. Also, without consumer input, user identity with service can deteriorate; and inappropriate use can occur. Perhaps it should be added that, as in the management of other affairs, the consumer wants in—a valid reason for involvement in its own right. There is no national means of providing the consumer the assistance he needs to become a positive force for improving the nation's health care services, nor do the means now exist for bringing the consumer and provider together to work jointly for improvements.

A number of the recommendations bear on the problem of decision making, involvement and education for this purpose.

> Any board or group set up to advise policy-making officials at any level of government must provide for consumer representation to protect and present the the interests and needs of the consumer. In addition, executive committees, subcommittees, and ad hoc committees of such board or groups should have a significant number of consumer representatives as members. Federal agencies involved in planning, delivering and purchasing health services must make provisions in budget for special orientation programs for new members of policy-making groups, including the consumer representatives on such groups.
>
> State and local agencies as well as nongovernmental agencies involved in planning for, delivering and paying for health services should be required to make provisions for orientation and training of policy-making groups, with special emphasis on consumer representatives.

Still with focus on the consumer, the Task Force underscored the desirability of instructing users of services on their rights and benefits and how to best use available services.

> Programs of health education, provided they meet adequate standards set by the Federal Government, should be considered integral components of any health care service and therefore included in the budget of such service. All agencies and institutions providing health services that receive Federal support must provide continuing programs of health education to their consumers.
>
> State Medicaid programs should be required to undertake educational efforts designed to: improve recip-

ients' use of the Medicaid program; improve the health of Medicaid recipients through preventive education; improve providers' use of the program, and provide for greater participation by provider and consumer in the planning, implementation, and evaluation of the program.

HEALTH CARE IN THE SLUMS [2]

It is laboring the obvious to stress that social conditions—housing, poverty, diet—have an enormous influence on health. Yet physicians who work in poor neighborhoods are unable to alter the conditions which cause much of what they must treat. And in trying to cure the symptoms, they work under additional, more subtle, handicaps. Whether any person will seek, accept, and follow treatment is dependent to a surprisingly large degree upon his beliefs and habits, not to mention his confidence in and understanding of his physician. Almost all doctors now practicing are from the middle class, and their education does little to prepare them for the realities of life in the slums, let alone the conceptions and misconceptions that may be firmly planted in the minds of their patients. Communication between physicians and even their middle-class patients is notoriously poor, between them and members of minority groups and other poor people with little education, it is probably far worse than they realize. The result is that medical care is often ineffective: medication is not taken as prescribed, diets are not followed, patients are afraid to ask questions or describe symptoms or give full histories.

In order to provide effective service, all those involved in delivering health care need to know something about the people they serve. A Carnegie Corporation grant to the OEO [Office of Economic Opportunity] supported Dr. Martin

[2] From "Extreme Remedies Are Very Appropriate for Extreme Diseases; American Health Care in Crisis." *Carnegie Quarterly.* 18:6-7. Summer '70. Reprinted by permission of the Carnegie Corporation of New York.

Luther King, Jr., Health Center in the south Bronx [a low-income area of New York City] enabled the Center to engage a sensitive cultural anthropologist, Alan Harwood. Under his supervision, eight people recruited from the neighborhood visited selected households twice a month for a period of a year, observing families and questioning them about health practices and illnesses as they occurred and participating in their lives—helping them with welfare problems, baby-sitting, hearing about and recording at first hand the day-to-day life in the community. The result is a valuable body of information on a fairly representative sample of the population, including standard demographic information as well as important facts about living conditions, diet, beliefs and practices about health, and relationships with the Health Center. Since the 45,000 people living in the neighborhood are mostly black and Puerto Rican, information was collected from both groups, revealing facts that have important implications for medical care.

Physicians often prescribe a drug to be taken with or after each meal, on the assumption that the patient will receive three doses a day approximately six hours apart. In the south Bronx, it turns out that people eat an average of 2.2 meals a day. (This does not include snacks such as pie or cake and soft drinks, which are consumed often.) Furthermore, the foods commonly eaten differ greatly from those of a middle-class white population, and standard therapeutic diets are generally unrealistic. Among black adults, for example, 46 per cent of the meat intake is pork, which makes it improbable that many would adhere to a low-cholesterol or low-fat diet unless realistic alternatives were provided. Among Puerto Ricans, salad is a very common and highly valued dietary item, and *sofrito,* a sauce containing tomatoes along with garlic, onions, and other spices, is a regular accompaniment to rice and meat. To restrict Puerto Ricans to a conventional bland diet is to prohibit those staples. One of the practical outgrowths of the Harwood team's research is two series of diets—low-calorie, bland, low-fat, etc.—one suitable for southern and one for Caribbean cuisine.

A more difficult problem relates to common understandings or misunderstandings about medical terms and conditions. In the terminology of many blacks in the neighborhood, for example, "high blood" is used to mean too much blood, "low blood" to mean too little blood, or anemia. If a patient is told that he has both high blood pressure and anemia he cannot believe it, since the two are mutually exclusive according to his own system of classification. The results of this kind of misunderstanding are obvious: the patient may not only refuse to take the medications prescribed but worse, lose confidence in his physician, since he finds the dual diagnosis completely inconsistent and therefore proof of the doctor's incompetence.

The potentialities for misunderstanding are of course multiplied when doctor and patient speak different languages. As another practical application of the Harwood research, the Health Center is now training Spanish-speaking medical assistants in translating and history-eliciting techniques.

Crucial to a patient's relationship to his doctor, and hence to his following a prescribed regimen, is whether the doctor fulfills the patient's expectation of how a doctor should behave, what he should do. Patients in the south Bronx (and probably everywhere) expect two basic things when they consult a physician: information and a "good" physical.

When the doctor makes a diagnosis (except in the case of a terminal illness, when some patients do not want to be told either the diagnosis or prognosis), the patient always wants to be told the name of the illness and basic information about it—the causes, effect on daily life, and how treatment helps or cures. The "good" physical consists of two things. First, the doctor must touch the patient—listen to the heart, for example. Merely taking a history and then prescribing medicine never constitutes a good physical. Second, any tests called for must be made relevant to the symptoms; if someone complains of stomach pains and is sent to have blood drawn, he wants to know what the tests have to do with his complaint.

Not surprisingly, considering the multitudinous opportunities for misunderstanding and doubt, Mr. Harwood's researchers found that few residents of the neighborhood take medicine as prescribed; they generally err in the direction of taking too little for too short a time. If the patient feels sleepy as a result of the medication, he reduces the dosage; when symptoms are relieved, medication is stopped. The patient then tends to share the excess tablets with sick friends or relatives.

Clearly these and other problems which reflect a less than satisfactory relationship—generally an authoritarian one—between doctor and patient are subtle and difficult to overcome. But better understanding should result in better communication. Mr. Harwood makes his findings available to the Health Center staff through a variety of formal and informal means and conducts in-service courses for pediatricians and internists, family health workers, and nurses on the Center's staff. Over the long run, however, the best hope appears to be strengthening medical education so that physicians will gain a better understanding of the cultural and psycho-social milieus in which they will work.

Mr. Harwood believes that there are two "teachable moments" in the life of the medical student—the times when he is most open to new ideas or a new orientation. One is during his first year of medical school. Mr. Harwood emphasizes that training in the social sciences during that year should be given a solid block of time and that the medical schools must make it clear that they consider them fully as important as the work in, say, anatomy or physiology. The second period, he believes, comes at the start of the internship. During the course of his four years of medical school the student has in most cases become "scientized" and tends to look at a patient

as a mass of symptoms. The change to a new educational setting provides a good opportunity to introduce a new view of
the patient as a total human being rooted in the totality of
his life.

HEALTH CARE GOES INTO THE STREETS [3]

The existence of a health gap in the United States is widely accepted. Despite the expression of concern by several
Presidents, it is still growing. Criteria such as infant and
maternal mortality, used to gauge a nation's delivery of
health care, show that the United States' ratings are shocking-
ly poor. In addition, skyrocketing prices have made health
care inaccessible to the poor and crippling for the middle
class.

New Health-Delivery System Needed

New ways to deliver health care are sorely needed. One
attempt has been launched by the Office of Economic Opportunity in its design of neighborhood health-center care for
the poor.

According to Dr. Thomas Bryant, associate director for
health affairs of OEO, the centers are bringing superior care
to the poor; moreover, they may point the way to a radical
revision of the nation's health-delivery system itself.

OEO statistics show that more than 23 million poor
people and an additional 13 million medically needy reside
in the United States. Health care normally provided to them,
inadequate as it is, has been permeated as well with a stigma
of charity. To replace it, OEO designed the neighborhood
centers primarily as a research undertaking. But to the slum
dweller, the centers have made possible a level of care that
just was not available before.

So far, 49 health centers, 13 of which are in rural areas, are
being funded in 23 states. But OEO asserts that more centers

[3] From article by Jeanne Bockel, staff writer. *Science News*. 97:276-7. Mr. 14,
'70. Reprinted, with permission from *Science News*, the weekly news magazine
of science and the applications of science, copyright 1970 by Science Service, Inc.

re needed because, if they were fully functional, they would
e sufficient to provide care for a million persons, and OEO
s seeking the funds for more.

The Neighborhood Health Centers emphasize family
medicine and serve everyone in the target area who is living
at the poverty level. They are tailor-made to the needs of the
community. As Dr. Bryant says, "It would be of no service to
have an English-speaking doctor in a Spanish-American community." In a city, he says, the center may deliver its services
to a community; in rural areas, a group of counties may be
served. But in either case, a well-organized center can provide
services for a population ranging from 10,000 to 30,000.

The largest center, the Watts center in the Los Angeles
ghetto, serves about 30,000 people, and employs about 40 to
50 physicians of all specialties. The physicians are divided
into teams that include about 4 to 5 doctors, 8 to 10 nurses,
social workers, family health workers and other paramedical
personnel. Each team serves many families and is able to accomplish what one physician never could. On the other hand,
in smaller centers, only 3 or 4 physicians, who practice basic
medicine, may be employed.

Services are provided on an outpatient basis and the
patient receives comprehensive services as preventive health,
diagnostic services, at-home care for chronic illness, rehabilitation, dental care, mental health services, drugs and ap-
pliances, and ambulance service.

If the patient needs hospital care, that too is arranged by
the center. His personal physician continues his medical
responsibility for the patient during hospitalization.

The emphasis, however, is on family medicine and the
patient is seen not only as an individual but as a member of
the family. Many health problems are related to family problems, and such issues as drinking problems, overcrowded conditions and whether both parents are working are explored
by the health team.

The Health Center

The health center provides the members of its staff th**
opportunity to deliver health services in a new social climate
Each center has a direct link to a hospital in the community
usually a teaching hospital, and all physicians have staff ap
pointments at the hospital.

The OEO centers are supported for a year or so by OE**
grants, but are also designed to use all sources of healt**
funds, encompassing Federal, state and local programs. Med
ical insurance payments are channeled through the center
as are payments for services to persons enrolled in Medicare
It is hoped that eventually Medicaid alone will be sufficien
to support the centers. But many states will not use Medicai**
funds for ambulatory care. This increases the cost of Medi
caid because it encourages even the best-intentioned physi**
cian to put the patient in a hospital. Dr. Bryant stresses tha
Medicaid must begin to support ambulatory care becaus**
"hospitalization costs money." This is a realization that i
already reflected in presidential policy; the support of hos
pital construction rather than ambulatory facilities was a**
issue in President Nixon's veto of the controversial Health
Education, and Welfare appropriations bill.

Dr. Bryant anticipates that Neighborhood Health Cen**
ters ultimately will operate without OEO subsidy, as the**
strengthen their resources through integrating other source**
of funds and services.

Although it is not universally accepted that the center**
have as yet been successful—any effort to extend them beyond
the poverty level is sure to be resisted—Dr. Bryant contend**
that a few points have been proved. He says that in ghettos
where there is no health care system, centers are the answer**
In areas where there are active public health centers with
group practice, however, then the answer may be to build on
this. "We can't say we've got a model and can spread i**
around," he says.

A second proven point, he says, is that people and institutions can be brought together to focus on the problem. City governments, the poor, physicians and public health workers have willingly joined in helping to provide health care to poor populations, he says.

The impact of success, claims Dr. Bryant, cannot be measured in two or three years. "It would take twenty years of practicing good preventive medicine before that can be done." But some measure of success is already being seen. In Denver, for instance, he believes the center is responsible for the fact that patients are not missing as many days at work, and lengths of hospitalization have decreased.

The Role of the Office of Economic Opportunity

If OEO's role is to prepare the system for universal health insurance by bringing about the necessary changes in the health care system, the next step, according to Dr. Bryant, is to move into preventive medicine outside the nation's ghettos.

Episodic health care for preventive medicine must be practiced. OEO can bring about this change by next entering the hospital outpatient departments and then into the hospitals themselves. Last summer [1969], OEO made sizable grants to four municipal hospital outpatient departments serving up to 200,000 persons, and hopes to expand the program to 5 to 10 cities in the next year.

ORGANIZING HEALTH CARE [4]

The supply of health manpower has not kept pace with the growth in the population or with the increased need for medical care. Moreover, present plans for more professional health schools hardly scratch the surface of need.

We are already in a crisis of supply, and that crisis would be compounded twice if poverty were eliminated overnight.

[4] From *The Health of the Poor*, by Irvin Block, medical affairs writer. (Pamphlet no 435) Public Affairs Committee, Inc. 381 Park Ave. S. New York 10016. '69. p 12-18. Reprinted by permission.

Thus, the question of adequate health care for the poor is more than a matter of educating the poor or of providing them with the money to buy care, or even of finding a way to eliminate poverty altogether. It is inextricably linked with the question of organizing health care.

How do you organize so as to accomplish this greater productivity with limited personnel, and yet provide a high degree of personal attention? How do you organize for the comprehensive approach, one that keeps in touch with the whole individual, his family and community, and makes available to him the whole range of specialized medical skills? How do you organize a health facility that doesn't wait to be called, but goes out seeking the community's health needs?

Some medical economists say that such questions are equally important for all America, not just for its poor. Even among the well-to-do, they say, there are few who truly get comprehensive, quality-controlled care. Medical services for the affluent, fragmented in various private offices, may be no less piecemeal than the various hospital specialty clinics that serve the poor, and are just as lacking in overall direction and informed management. All health care must be reorganized, they say, not just that for the poor.

Others, while agreeing on the need for a major reorganization of health care for everybody, do not feel that a special effort for the poor must wait. They feel that a unique opportunity for demonstrating such reorganization exists in the poverty areas, where the need is more urgent and there is less commitment to existing means of distributing health services. Such demonstrations can provide "ghetto medicine" that is high in quality, broad in distribution, offering an example of effective organization to all communities regardless of status.

Neighborhood Health Centers

There are a few such demonstrations in existence, such as neighborhood health centers made possible by grants from he Office of Economic Opportunity. They offer the model of the "comprehensive community health center." They are not all exactly the same, differing in their style with differences in communities and with the bents of their leadership. However, they share an approach that, in the opinion of this writer and of many public health experts who have concerned themselves for years with the problems of poverty and health care, offers great promise for better medicine for more people. They combine a number of ideas that have served America well: community organization, social settlement work, local self-rule, and efficient management of a team of experts.

The approach is best illustrated by describing the operations of the pioneer program at Columbia Point in Boston, begun in December 1965. In this venture, the department of preventive medicine at Tufts University School of Medicine undertook to perform the role of family doctor and health manager for a community of some 6,000 persons living in low-income housing built on a former city dump in Boston Harbor. The range of services provided by the center, as described by its chief organizer, Dr. Jack Geiger are:

Emergency, sick child and well child, sick adult and adult health screening, home medical care and home nursing, health education, psychiatric services, social work, community organization, laboratory, pharmacy, ambulance and patient transportation, specialty consultation, prenatal care, and close ties with teaching hospitals and consultants for hospitalization or special needs.

To begin with, everybody in Columbia Point is eligible for care. Eligibility is a matter of residence; this avoids the humiliating procedures of proving poverty. Further, the Center is *in* the community, within walking distance of every resident, and it is open twenty-four hours a day. This disposes of the barriers of time and distance.

A satellite hospital clinic? Not at all! The Columbia Point Center is manned by people—from physicians to floor scrubbers—who work there full time, on salary. This is their only job, their main responsibility. There are no Lady Bountifuls,

no doctors donating a few harassed hours a week to charity
Indeed, the Center staff and patients see the Center as the
source of the community's health care, with the hospitals as
its satellites, to be used as needed.

In Dr. Geiger's words:

It is the Health Center that definitively arranges with its satel
lite hospital . . . and with a network of consultants and other spe
cialty facilities in Boston, for the things it does not provide itself
hospitalization and consultation in the important but less fre
quently used specialties. To "arrange definitively" means, to us
to take responsibility, and so we see to it that appointments are
made, that patients are transported to other facilities and back to
Columbia Point where necessary, and that the resulting data from
other sources are incorporated into Columbia Point Health Cen
ter records, so that continuity is preserved.

Personal, continuous, concerned care—that is the watch
word at Columbia Point, in sharp contrast to the piecemeal
impersonal service that characterizes the present hospita
clinics. The basic care-giving unit is the family health car
group, a team consisting of one or two internists, one or two
pediatricians, several community health nurses, several socia
workers, and "nonprofessional" community health aides
Each Columbia Point family is assigned to one of these teams
whose job it is to know the family's problems with an inti
macy and thoroughness far deeper than ever attained by the
old-fashioned single family doctor. Moreover, this team car
bring a range of skills to bear on the family's problems tha
the single family doctor could never hope to muster. The
team takes responsibility for the family's health, not merely
its sickness, and not only when symptoms appear. The intern
ists supervise the health needs of the family adults, the pedia
tricians of the children, both summoning specialists when
needed. The nurses implement the medical care at the Center
and in the home. Social workers follow the family's economic
and social problems. The work of these professionals is ex
tended and amplified by community health aides, a new clas
of health worker.

Community Health Aides

The work of the community health aides bears special mention. Many experts in medical care are recognizing the importance of developing paramedical aides—nonprofessional assistants to doctors, nurses, and social workers—as an answer to the shortage of professionally trained people. Such persons can be trained to carry out the more routine and time-consuming functions of the doctors, nurses, and social workers. However, in a community health center like Columbia Point, such aides perform functions that go far beyond that of providing extra arms and legs for hard-pressed professionals. Recruited locally, they bring an intimate knowledge of the community, its ways, problems, and culture, to the treatment team. They help fill in communication gaps between the professionals and the neighborhood. They help demonstrate to the people of the community that this is indeed *their* health care facility. Very often, they suggest to doctors and nurses better ways of getting things done, both medically and socially.

And just as important, the development of these aides makes needed jobs and trains important skills, providing a direct economic lift out of the poverty trap for many people. At Columbia Point, about 40 per cent of the staff is composed of community residents who have been trained for special jobs. Moreover, these jobs are negotiable; many so trained have moved to other jobs out of Columbia Point. Thus, the Center has brought outward economic mobility as well as health care—a many-faceted intervention in the general problem of poverty.

The community is further involved in the work of the health center through the organization of a local Health Association. This group acts as a sort of local board of governors, participating in making policy and plans.

Measuring Success

How successful has the venture been? Only ten months after the Center opened its doors, more than 80 per cent of

Columbia Point residents used its services at least once. More than two hundred persons a day are now being seen. In two years the rate of hospitalization in the community dropped 80 per cent, the proportion of families who postponed medical care was reduced to 5 per cent from its previous 23 per cent, and the number of residents who have had a recent medical checkup was doubled.

As yet, the Columbia Point project has not served as a teaching facility for doctors, mainly because it wished to break the traditional pattern whereby the poor received their medical care from the part-time services of medical trainees and instructors. This was essential in winning the community's confidence. Also the leadership wanted to study and learn how to teach in such a setting. The utilization of medical students at all levels is an important part of the future plans for these kinds of projects. The comprehensive health center offers opportunities for training doctors in family care and community work that the hospital setting cannot provide. Medical interns who spend a portion of their training terms in such a community center are bound to have a stronger orientation toward family health care than those whose internships are spent only in hospitals. Further, an association with teaching is needed to help keep the health center in the mainstream of the medical world.

Other Programs

Columbia Point is not unique. It is cited here because it was the first of its kind. The Office of Economic Opportunity provides assistance to 47 other Comprehensive Health Services projects. Thirty-four are urban, and 13 are rural. The Children's Bureau and the Public Health Service provide aid to other projects. The range of experimentation is wide, as it needs to be in the uncharted area of better health care for the poor. Some programs follow lines pioneered by Columbia Point. Some are under hospital auspices. There are even a few trial projects in which groups of private

doctors have contracted to provide comprehensive care to
groups of poor patients. In some instances the OEO has
used its funds to enable existing group health plans to
service the poor on the same basis as paying members.

These projects are directed toward goals that make medical sense: comprehensive and preventive care, quality control,
better and more efficient use of our scarce doctors and nurses,
and family-oriented personal medicine.

Many see the neighborhood health center as a solution
to more than "ghetto medicine." Dr. Geiger says:

I am seriously suggesting that the hospital as we now know it
is an obsolete and ineffective institution for ambulatory care, and
that hospitals for the future should be vastly different—in effect,
intensive care units for patients with critical and complex illness,
and a more modest section . . . for ambulatory patients requiring
bed care and for completely ambulatory patients requiring complex specialty resources. The hub of the medical care universe
would be a network of comprehensive community health centers.
I believe this model is just as appropriate for middle-income groups
as for the disadvantaged, and should not be restricted to the poor—
but in this initial effort, the poor, with their greatest needs, should
have the first priority.

V. SOCIETY'S VALUES AND ITS HEALTH

EDITOR'S INTRODUCTION

If there were ever any doubt that the changing value of a society have a bearing on medical issues, the revolu tionary changes in the public attitude toward abortion ar proof of a close interrelationship. Once an almost unmen tionable subject, abortion is today an issue for open, anc serious, national debate. Although most states presentl' prohibit abortions, except to save the mother's life, this yea more than a million women will have them. Under pressur from some women's groups, clergymen, doctors, and socia workers, some states have already changed their laws t make abortions possible under certain circumstances. Othe states are considering some liberalization.

This section examines some specific health problem facing the American people today. Some of these, lik cancer, are purely physical diseases. Some, like abortior overeating, and anxiety are not physical diseases at a but medical problems connected with society's values. Som like heart disease and venereal disease, are both physica diseases and direct reflections on how a society's changin values affect the health of the people in that society. Th range of contemporary sociomedical controversy, however, i far too widespread to encompass within this section, for i includes subjects as diverse as air and water pollution, gene ic control of heredity, drug addiction, and fluoridation.

The initial articles in this section deal with aspects c abortion. The first, an excerpt from Senior Scholastic, e amines the legal and moral issues behind the abortion cor troversy. The second, by Dr. Denis Cavanagh, argues again: the increasing liberalization of abortion laws.

Next, an excerpt from *Time* describes the surprising increase in venereal disease in the past decade—surprising because venereal diseases can easily be treated by antibiotics today.

The fourth article, from *U.S. News & World Report*, examines the findings of a two-year study of heart disease undertaken at the request of the U.S. Government. The following two articles examine various aspects of the fight against cancer in the United States. In the first, the outlines of the mammoth task of conquering cancer are given. The second examines the possible connection between cancer and viruses.

Can members of the wealthiest society in the history of the world be malnourished? Yes, say nutritionists. Many Americans are not only malnourished; they can be, paradoxically, overweight at the same time. Mary Bralove, staff reporter of the *Wall Street Journal*, shows us how in the next excerpt. Freelance writer William Barry Furlong writes next of stress and its prime symptom, the headache, perhaps the most common malady today. Then, William Gerber of *Editorial Research Reports* studies the pervasive inroads stress makes in the lives of people in a modern industrial society. Finally, Dr. Alexander Leaf, Jackson Professor of Clinical Medicine at Harvard University, describes how new advances in medicine pose some difficult choices for society—for example, who is going to be saved and who is not.

ABORTION: THE MORAL DILEMMA [1]

Is it right to end a woman's pregnancy before a baby is born? Throughout history, people have given a wide variety of answers. The ancient Greek philosopher Aristotle approved of abortion in certain cases. Many early Jewish and Christian leaders disapproved, saying only God had a right

[1] From "Abortion Tumult." *Senior Scholastic.* 96:7-8. My. 4, '70. Reprinted permission of Scholastic Magazines, Inc., from *Senior Scholastic,* © 1970 by Scholastic Magazines, Inc.

to decide the fate of a child after conception. In Englan
and America, the question was widely regarded until rela
tively recently as a matter for religious decision. It was no
until the nineteenth century that the first abortion law
were passed. These made abortion illegal except unde
special circumstances—for example, to save the mother's life

An estimated one million abortions are performed i
the United States every year. Only about 8,000 of these ar
legal. When performed under sterile conditions by a qual
fied doctor, an abortion in early pregnancy is usually
safe, routine operation. When performed incompetently, i
can result in severe injury or even death. Anywhere fror
500 to 1,000 women die in the United States every year as
result of illegal abortions. Some authorities believe this i
the major cause of death among pregnant women today.

In recent years, pressure has mounted for changes i
abortion laws. England, Hungary, the Soviet Union, Japar
and a number of other nations permit abortion at a woman
request. In this country, Maryland, North Carolina, Colc
rado, and other states have modified earlier laws to mak
them more permissive. They generally allow abortions unde
certain specific conditions. For example: when there is
risk a baby will be abnormal; when the mother is unwe
and under sixteen; when pregnancy threatens the physic;
or mental health of the mother; when pregnancy is th
result of rape. In thirty-seven states, however, abortion
allowed only to save the mother's life.

. . . [In March 1970] Hawaii became the first U.S. state t
permit abortion "on demand." Hawaii now requires onl
that the abortion be done in the first four or five montl
of pregnancy. The woman must have lived in Hawaii fc
ninety days—to prevent a flood of women from other stat(
from coming to Hawaii for an abortion.

New York has also changed its law to permit abortio
upon a woman's request, during the first twenty-four weel
of pregnancy. The New York law does not require that th

woman be a New York resident. Legislators in Maryland and Arizona have also been considering proposals to legalize abortion completely.

The arguments for and against changes in abortion laws go straight to basic questions about life itself. The Roman Catholic Church, along with some other religions, strongly opposes abortion. The official Roman Catholic position is that the fetus (unborn child) is a living human being with a soul. In the Roman Catholic Church's view, the deliberate destruction of the fetus amounts to murder.

Those who oppose legalizing abortion argue that men should not take it upon themselves to decide who shall be born and who shall not. . . . [In 1969], this argument helped bring defeat of a reform bill in New York State. A dramatic speech by Assemblyman Martin Ginsberg, who is crippled from polio, helped defeat the bill. He objected to a proposal that would have allowed abortion if the baby might be abnormal. "What this bill says is that those who are malformed or abnormal have no reason to be part of our society," he said.

Other opponents of legalizing abortion call it "a prelude to trading lives." One lawyer put it this way: "Once you start to lower the value of life in any form, you lower the value of life in all forms."

Defenders of abortion disagree. "A fetus is no more a human than an acorn is an oak," asserts Dr. Robert E. Hall of Columbia University. A fetus is not able to live independent of the mother until some time after twenty weeks, he says.

Outright repeal of antiabortion laws is now backed by several religious and other groups. These include the American Baptist Convention, the American Jewish Congress, and the American Public Health Association.

Many of those who favor reform argue that abortion is a matter that should be settled by the individual woman and her doctor. "No law tells me if I can amputate a leg.

And no law should govern whether I am to perform an abortion," says Dr. Carl Goldmark, a director of the Association for the Study of Abortion.

Women's rights organizations and many civil right groups argue that women should have the right to decide whether or not to bear children. They say most of the anti-abortions laws were passed by all-male legislatures. Several recent court decisions have supported—at least in part— the view that many antiabortion laws deny women their rights.

"There is nothing worse than an unwilling mother and an unwilling child," asserts State Senator D. Clinton Dominick (New York). "It leads to divorce. It leads to broken homes [and] neglected children."

The reformers also argue that it is the poor women who have to pay. A middle or upper income woman can often go to another country or to a private hospital for a legal abortion. But these safe abortions are not available to poor women, the reformers say. Poor women often go to unqualified abortionists working under makeshift, unsanitary conditions. The reformers point out that the death rate in New York City for illegal abortions is ten times higher among black and Puerto Rican women than among white women.

A DOCTOR LOOKS AT ABORTION [2]

At one point in the [International Conference on Abortion held in Washington, D.C., in 1967 and attended by proponents and opponents], a Senator asked me if I ever felt there was an indication for therapeutic abortion. I replied in the affirmative. I believe there is a place for therapeutic abortion, and there is no doubt that it may be necessary to kill a fetus to save the life of the mother. But this situation is very rare in modern obstetrical practice

[2] From "Reforming the Abortion Laws: A Doctor Looks at the Case," by Dr. Denis Cavanagh. *America*. 122:406-11. Ap. 18, '70. Reprinted with permission from *America,* April 18, 1970. All rights reserved. © 1970 America Press, Inc., 106 West 56 Street, New York 10019.

I think there is no justification for the statement that mothers die because we do not have a liberal law in the state of Missouri. I am director of the Obstetrics Service at the St. Louis City Hospital. This is a hospital that serves the underprivileged almost exclusively and where one would expect a high maternal mortality rate. But over the period July 1, 1966, to July 1, 1968, we had 5,102 deliveries without a single maternal death. This compares very well with the national maternal mortality rate of approximately 3 per 10,000 live births. During this two-year period only one therapeutic abortion was considered necessary to save the life of a mother.

I submit therefore that there is no evidence that liberalization of the abortion law in accordance with American Law Institute recommendations will reduce the maternal mortality in the state of Missouri or in any other state.

It was also stated by the proponents for liberalization in Missouri that the typical patient requesting abortion is aged twenty-five, has had more than three previous pregnancies and is married. But if you look at the report on the first year of experience with the liberalized law in the state of Colorado, you will note that although the law was supposed to be designed primarily to assist the hard-pressed mother of several children whose mental or physical health was threatened by another pregnancy, only 138 of 407 women who received therapeutic abortions (that is about one third) were married, and 56.5 per cent of the women had had no previous pregnancies. Only 22.4 per cent of the women who had therapeutic abortions performed had three or more living children. . . .

Every reasonable person is concerned about the delivery of an abnormal baby, and so a great deal of pressure has been developed in this area. Immediately the questions arise, of course: How affected is affected? What is a minimal defect and what is a major defect? Here are some figures on the 1964 rubella epidemic from Harvey and Thompson. Dr. Harvey is from the State Department of Health in

Indiana; Dr. Thompson is in the Department of Obstetrics and Gynecology at the Indiana University School of Medicine. These men gave evidence before the Committee to Study the Indiana Abortion Law. They pointed out that in the 1964 epidemic the number of German measles cases was approximately ten times the number of cases seen in a normal year, yet only 43 anomalies were found among 280 babies born of women who had developed rubella during the first trimester of pregnancy. . . .

Another point seldom mentioned is the fact that rubella vaccine will be in full use before the next rubella epidemic. By the use of this vaccine rubella should disappear from the United States as a significant problem, just as poliomyelitis has disappeared since the introduction of the polio vaccines. And remember that rubella is by far the most common cause of fetal abnormalities at this time. The proponents are well-informed people who know that this indication will disappear with the vaccine, but they selectively forget it because it weakens their case. And yet, does anyone here really believe that once the vaccine has been proved effective the legislatures will quickly repeal the anachronistic law?

Normal Or Defective Babies?

There are other uncommon causes of fetal anomalies, but even with modern methods it is usually impossible to tell for certain when a child will be born with certain defects. A prediction can usually only be based on probabilities. Thus a significant number of normal children will be killed to prevent the birth of one having what may be only a minor birth defect. After all, what is a birth defect? Adolf Hitler believed that being Jewish was a defect of birth. Some scientists interested in preserving only the best of our human species believe it is a defect to be too stupid, too tall, too short, too white or too black.

Where life or death is the issue, it is not unreasonable to insist that a duty is owed to the living but as yet unborn

tus. If the doctor has erred in his diagnosis, has acted
unreasonably or is engaged in a thriving abortion business,
there is no appeal from his decision, no rehearing and no
retrial. His judgment is final, conclusive and irrevocable.
There is no tomorrow for the aborted child.

The so-called humane provision regarding birth defects,
unless analyzed carefully, may very well result in a signi-
cant change in the moral and legal philosophy upon which
our culture is based. Once it has been determined that life
can be taken away for a birth defect, it may be taken away
for other reasons. After all, the true description of the
procedure with regard to the presumably deformed child is
not therapeutic abortion, because there is nothing therapeutic in it for the baby. It is at the best fetal euthanasia.

We may learn something from the English experience.
Those who were pushing for a liberalized abortion law
in Britain three years ago are now pushing for euthanasia
and a Euthanasia Bill was only defeated in the House of
Lords by 61 votes to 40 in 1969.

How can we call abortion "humanitarian" when dis-
missing a presumably deformed fetus? This sounds good
until you try to put yourself in the position of that fetus.
It is difficult for any obstetrician, after all, to decide whether
the child, even though deformed, does not have a right to be
born, for the deformities may be minimal.

The New Jersey Supreme Court has eloquently answered
this question in the affirmative in the 1967 case of Gleitman
Cosgrove (1945-49 N.J. 22). The court declared:

> It is basic to the human condition to seek life and to hold on
> to it however heavily burdened. If Jeffrey [the baby born de-
> formed, whose parents brought suit] could have been asked as to
> whether his life should be snuffed out before his full term of gesta-
> tion could run its course, our felt intuition of human nature tells
> us that he would almost surely choose life with defects as against no
> life at all.

Leaving aside all the theological and legal arguments, as

Theocritus said, "for the living there is hope but for th
dead there is none."

The crux of the moral and legal debate over abortion i
in essence, the right of the woman to determine whethe
or not she should bear a particular child versus the rigl
of the child to life. The most vigorous proponents of lil
eralization talk about the fetus as "a blob of protoplasm
and feel it has no right to life until it has reached a ce:
tain stage of development. This is given variously as fro»
12 weeks to 28 weeks of intrauterine life, and some appa
ently feel it has no right to life until after full-term deliver
On the other hand, the most vigorous opponents of lil
eralization maintain that the fetus is human from the tim
of conception, and so interruption of pregnancy cannot b
justified from the time of fertilization.

I have some doubt about whether the fetus can b
recognized as a separate human being from the time of fe
tilization. But it certainly seems logical that from the stag
of differentiation, after which neither twinning nor recon
bination will occur, the fetus implanted in the uterin
wall deserves respect as a human life. If we take the d«
finition of life as being said to be present when an organis:
shows evidence of individual animate existence, I thin
that certainly from the blastocyst stage the fetus qualifie
for respect. It is alive because it has the ability to reproduc
dying cells. It is human because it can be distinguishe
from other nonhuman species, and once implanted in th»
uterine wall it requires only nutrition and time to develo
into one of us.

If it contains an intrinsic genetic defect, or if it is de
prived of nutrition and time, it becomes a dead huma
fetus. I think that this is a reasonable, philosophical co:
clusion based on biological knowledge. It recognizes tha
human development is a single continuous process fro:
implantation of the fertilized ovum in the uterine wall t
the achievement of adult personhood. It seems quite i:
rational, even if convenient, to choose a given point in th:

biologic continuum—e.g., the appearance of the heartbeat, or the feeling of movements, or even expulsion from the uterus—as the beginning of human life. It seems evident that the fetus is only different from you and me in that it has not yet been given the time to develop its whole potential.

VD: A NATIONAL EMERGENCY[3]

The global outbreak of syphilis and gonorrhea spawned by World War II came as no surprise to the medical world. Over the past five centuries, there had been massive flare-ups of venereal disease—the worst of them during wartime. But the World War II epidemic was cut short by the 1945 discovery that both diseases could be cured by penicillin. The numbers of new cases reported annually in the United States declined through the 1950s and early 1960s, and venereologists hoped that the twin scourges would soon be wiped out.

In recent years, however, venereal disease has been making a comeback. In 1965, Dr. William J. Brown of the U.S. Center for Disease Control declared that an estimated 550,000 Americans under twenty were annually contracting either syphilis or gonorrhea. Reported cases of syphilis in the past year have risen by 55 per cent in New Jersey, 30 per cent in New York City. . . . [In July 1970] Dr. James McKenzie-Pollock of the American Social Health Association reported that there has been a "spectacular rise" in syphilis in the past five months and called for national emergency action to meet the problem.

Epidemiologists do not agree on the causes for VD's current upswing. Health authorities admit that the Vietnam conflict has had little impact on U.S. health. Many doctors believe that the preliminary victories of penicillin over VD were oversold, and that a false sense of security was created, especially among the young. Some blame the

[3] From article in *Time*. 96:36. Jl. 27, '70. Reprinted by permission from *Time*, The Weekly Newsmagazine; Copyright Time, Inc. 1970.

Pill, claiming that oral contraceptives are being widel used instead of condoms. But the use of condoms ha actually increased since 1960. Only one thing is certain no one can satisfactorily explain the current epidemic.

Massachusetts disease detectives, who rank among th best organized in the nation, say that prostitutes are t blame for only about 3 per cent of cases: "They usuall know how to take pretty good care of themselves." Mal homosexuality is blamed for 16 per cent and heterosexua free love for 81 per cent.

Untreated, syphilis goes through three principal phases The early stages may be marked at first by visible sores later by a rash, and are highly infectious for about a yea unless treated. The next is the "silent phase," when th disease is relatively noninfectious and can be detected onl by blood test. This may last several years, followed by th late stage, which can cause heart damage, blindness o general paralysis.

Gonorrhea is usually considered less serious, but is mor "catching." And it can be inapparent in a woman, whos only sign of infection may be a slight vaginal discharge– which might result from a multitude of other causes. A male victim is more likely to seek prompt medical help, a he will probably suffer a painful urethral discharge.

However they disagree on other matters, medical au thorities see an answer to VD epidemics in a combination of case reporting and contact tracing. But the U.S. Gov ernment spends only $6.3 million a year on case and contac finding; with money from the states and municipalities used mostly for education, the total spent on VD is les than $30 million. It seems likely that neither syphilis no gonorrhea will be eradicated until vaccines against them are prepared. But research on such preventive measures i even more starved of financial support than case finding and treatment.

THE "GOOD LIFE" VERSUS YOUR HEART [4]

Reprinted from *U.S. News & World Report.*

A new worldwide study of heart disease in human beings hows that living "the good life" in the United States and other advanced nations really is a way to early death for many people.

If you are "living it up" and want to cut your risk of heart trouble, you may have to change your entire way of life—diet, smoking, working and relaxing—say the health authorities who prepared the report.

Rigorous and far-reaching Government action also will be necessary, they say, if heart disease—the nation's No. 1 killer—is to be controlled.

These are the conclusions of 115 health experts after a two-year study undertaken at the request of the U.S. Government. The study was under direction of the American Heart Association, with funds from the Department of Health, Education, and Welfare. Twenty-nine national health groups participated.

Other highlights from the report:

One out of every 5 American men will develop heart disease before he reaches age sixty. In most cases a heart attack will be the first sign of trouble.

One victim in 4 will die within three hours of his first heart attack. Of those who survive, 1 in 10 will die a few weeks after an initial attack.

People who have had one heart attack are approximately five times as likely to die within five years after the event as people without known heart ailments.

Under age sixty-five, American men are three times as likely to die of coronary disease as women.

What Are the Causes?

The most common cause of heart trouble among adults in the United States and other advanced countries is **not**

[4] From article in *U.S. News & World Report.* 69:29. D. 28, '70.

located in the heart at all, the report points out. A con
dition called atherosclerosis, which results when layers o
fatty materials cause a thickening of the arteries, can lead to
strokes, kidney trouble and other serious ills besides hear
attacks.

A number of fatty materials called lipids may be to
blame for atherosclerosis. Of these, cholesterol is probably
the principal culprit, according to the report.

A study of twenty-two countries throughout the world
showed that where people consumed a lot of fat in meat or
butter and had a lot of cholesterol in their blood—as they
do in the affluent United States—they had a lot of hear
trouble, too.

The experts also found a direct relation between ciga
rette smoking and heart disease. The earlier you start ciga
rette smoking, the earlier you are risking coronary difficulty
the more cigarettes you smoke, the more likely you are to have
heart trouble.

People who are overweight, those who have high blood
pressure, those who do not exercise enough, and those who
live and work in tense surroundings also are listed as high
risk candidates for heart disease.

Each of these factors, taken alone, increases the likeli
hood of heart trouble. When they are combined, as they
would be in a person who eats a lot of fat, has high blood
pressure and smokes many cigarettes, the likelihood of heart
disease increases, the research findings show.

What Individuals Can Do

Once your arteries start to narrow and clog up, there
is not much that can be done to clear them, the experts
find. They say the facts "strongly indicate that major pro
gress in controlling atherosclerotic diseases is possible only
by primary prevention."

These steps are recommended:

Watch your diet. Use lean cuts of meat. Avoid solid
fats, such as butter, lard, suet, bacon. Avoid rich pastries,

andies and cakes. Avoid egg yolks. Instead use grains, ruits, vegetables, lean meats and fish.

Stop smoking cigarettes. Try cigars or a pipe if you nust smoke.

See a doctor. He can look for heart trouble, prescribe lrugs to ease high blood pressure and a diet to reduce holesterol and other fats in the blood. He can check for liabetes—which is highly dangerous to the heart—and may irge you to exercise and to lose excess fat.

What Government Can Do

The report also suggested some steps the Federal Government should take:

Promote the development and sale of leaner meat.

Stop using butterfat content as the pricing standard for lairy products.

Develop ways of reducing the solid-fat and cholesterol content of cheeses and bakery products.

Give high priority to "the elimination of cigarette smoking as a national habit."

THE WAR ON CANCER [5]

No affliction that man is heir to is quite so heavily freighted with dread and mystery as cancer. One reason for this is that, to many, the word itself is synonymous with death—and with protracted suffering. For no part of the human body is immune to cancer. The malignancy eats into nerve and muscle, bone and organ, blood and lymph alike; and it acquires an extra measure of terror because of the stealth with which it arises and because its deadly origins are inexplicably intertwined with the secret of life itself.

[5] From "The War on Cancer: Progress Report." *Newsweek*. 77:84-90. F. 22, '71. Copyright Newsweek, Inc. 1971. Reprinted by permission.

This year alone some 330,000 Americans will die c
cancer. Of the 200-odd million Americans now alive an
well, fully 25 per cent, or some 50 million, will one da
hear their doctors pronounce the dread diagnosis. Of thes
about 34 million will die, and even some of those who a
saved may not consider themselves lucky. Thousands wi
be disfigured by the therapists' attempts to excise or bur
away the malignancy. Other thousands will linger on, fc
months, for years, some for quite a few years. Perhaps th
cruelest truth of all is that of those doomed to die th:
year of cancer, 4,000 are children.

Faced with these grim statistics, it is small wonder tha
the United States Congress almost routinely designates th
National Cancer Institute to receive the biggest single slic
of Federal medical research funds, or that concerned ord
nary citizens . . . [in 1970] contributed $65 million to th
American Cancer Society. It is also small wonder that th
war against cancer has regularly enlisted the talents an
dedication of so many of the nation's most outstandin
scientists and researchers. What is new in the war agains
cancer is that this year [1971], for perhaps the first tim
in memory, there is in the making a dramatic concatenatio
of major scientific achievement on the one hand, and o
massive public commitment on the other.

The result is that despite the picture of almost ur
relieved gloom projected by the statistics, the war agains
cancer has entered a new and hopeful phase. There is n
cure in sight. That must be said at once. But scientifi
discoveries in recent years, months and even weeks hav
lifted the level of cancer research to a dramatic new plateau
And, coincidentally or not, the White House itself has calle
for a massive commitment of public funds. "The time ha
come in America," said President Richard M. Nixon in hi
State of the Union message . . . [in 1971], "when the sam
kind of concentrated effort that split the atom and took ma
to the moon should be turned toward conquering this drea
disease."

For the moment, the ultimate size and shape—not to mention the efficacy—of this kind of campaign are uncertain; this will probably remain so for some time, while partisans of both political parties maneuver for the credit and the limelight in what is to come. But it seems certain enough that something substantially beyond any past similar commitment will emerge. Meanwhile the war proceeds ever more encouragingly at almost every tactical salient—in the diagnostician's office, in the operating room, in the radiotherapists' chambers and, above all, in the laboratories of the quiet, patient and painstaking men whose researches into the mystery of life itself may one day solve the deathly riddle of the cancer cell that lurks there.

There is no lack of evidence that the new optimism is warranted. Just three decades ago, only one cancer patient in five had a chance of survival. Today the figure stands at nearly 40 per cent. In some forms of cancer, the survival rate has risen even more dramatically. Now 60 to 80 per cent of the female patients with breast cancer are being saved by the surgeon's knife. New advances in radiation therapy have drastically improved the chances of patients with Hodgkin's disease, a cancer of the lymph glands. Drug therapy is prolonging the lives of children with leukemia, and in some cases doctors are now even going so far as to pronounce their patients cured of this tragic killer.

THE VIRUS-CANCER MYSTERY [6]

For centuries, scientists have sought the cause of one of man's most baffling diseases—cancer. Today, evidence is rapidly accumulating that viruses, long known to cause cancer in animals, also may cause cancer in humans.

Two viruses appear to be prime suspects: Epstein-Barr virus (EBV) and herpes type 2. Recent research

[6] From "New Clues in the Virus-Cancer Mystery," by Clyde R. Goodheart, M.D., head of cancer virology studies at the Institute for Biomedical Research, and Barbara Goodheart, freelance writer. *Today's Health*. 48:32-5. Je. '70. *Today's Health* is copyrighted and published by the American Medical Association.

strengthens the link, suspected for several years, between EBV and Burkitt's tumor, a type of cancer seen chiefly in African children. EBV is consistently found in cells from Burkitt's tumor and is believed to cause the tumor only in persons who also have been infected with malaria. Curiously, the same virus apparently has caused infectious mononucleosis in persons in the United States, where malaria is virtually unknown.

Even newer evidence links herpes type 2 with cancer of the cervix (neck of the uterus), one of the most common types of cancer in women. Studies show that four out of five women with this disease have antibodies to herpes type 2, compared to only one in five who are free of the disease.

Both EBV and herpes type 2 belong to a group known as herpesviruses. Other herpesviruses cause chicken pox, cold sores, and other mild diseases, but do not appear in any way involved in cancer. Yet certain characteristics of the group as a whole strengthen the suspicion concerning EBV and herpes type 2. Several animal herpesviruses are known to cause cancer in animals. And herpesviruses can remain dormant in an animal or human for long periods. Researchers suspect that some eventually are "turned on" in some way, becoming capable of causing cancer.

Scientists feel they can apply their knowledge of viruses toward an eventual means of preventing or curing some forms of human cancer. They foresee development of vaccines to protect against cancer viruses, though this will take many years. And vaccines may not be the final answer to all types of human cancer. Other possibilities are drugs to inhibit cancer viruses permanently or drugs to strengthen the immune system, enabling the body to fight off cancer cells.

If viruses cause cancer, can we "catch" the disease from someone who has it? There is no reason to avoid contact with a cancer patient. Careful epidemiological studies have failed to show that cancer can spread from one person to another in the usual communicable disease pattern. Futhermore, an apparent link exists between certain chemicals and cancer, and between smoking and lung cancer. This could mean that viruses are not the only cause of cancer, or that an activating agent, such as chemicals present in cigarette smoke, may be required by some viruses if they are to cause cancer.

A virus is a tiny organism consisting of a molecule of genetic material (nucleic acid) surrounded by a protein coat. Unable to reproduce by itself, a virus takes on its only semblance of life when it invades a living cell.

Once inside a cell, a virus usually "orders" the cell to manufacture new viruses. Instead of functioning normally, the cell makes hundreds or thousands of virus particles, then dies. The new viruses enter nearby healthy cells and repeat the cycle. Typically, the body responds to the attack by producing two protective substances—interferon and antibodies. Interferon, manufactured in gradually increasing amounts soon after the infection begins, helps protect healthy cells from the virus. If interferon fails to stop the virus attack, the body may make antibodies—blood proteins that inactivate the virus and create permanent immunity in the individual.

An alternate type of virus-cell interaction is the one that most interests cancer researchers. If the virus does not use the cell for the production of new viruses, it loses its identity and becomes part of the cell's genetic information. Garbling the cell's genetic instructions, the virus calls for uncontrolled growth. The cell divides, passing new orders to new generations of cells. The result is cancer—uncontrolled growth of cells that refuse to stay within their allotted boundaries. . . .

Although most herpesviruses—including herpes simplex, which causes cold sores—do not seem in any way involved in cancer, researchers point out that the herpesvirus group differs from many other virus groups in three important ways:

1. Most known herpes cancer viruses cause cancer in the natural host, the animal in which they are found in nature. To date, many other known cancer viruses cause cancer only under artificial conditions—when injected in animals they do not normally infect.

2. Some herpesviruses are passed through the placenta; thus, they can infect an unborn child. This is important because, with one exception, all known cancer viruses cause cancer only when they infect newborn animals. (The exception is a monkey herpesvirus that causes cancer when injected into adult monkeys.)

3. Many animal and human herpesviruses have an unusual characteristic known as latency—the ability to survive in the natural host in a dormant form. Scientists suspect that a latent virus may be in a state of incomplete maturation. To reach maturity, it may require substances not immediately available or another factor, such as a temperature change. Once "turned on," it may be capable of causing cancer.

There is still no *proof* that viruses cause human cancer. But most scientists are proceeding on the assumption that proof soon will be established.

Preliminary steps are being taken toward vaccines to protect against EBV and herpes type 2. At Roswell Park Memorial Institute, Buffalo, New York, researchers are developing an experimental EBV vaccine using part of the protein coat of the virus, rather than weakened or killed virus, to minimize possible side effects.

Recent development of an experimental vaccine to protect chickens against Marek's disease—a cancer caused by a herpesvirus—may mean human herpesvirus vaccines will not be difficult to develop. Yet scientists emphasize that even if all experiments go perfectly, human vaccines will not be ready for public use for at least eight years. And many feel that vaccines will not be the final answer to all types of human cancer. Some cancer viruses may prove difficult to isolate and identify—steps which must precede vaccine development. Also the possibility still exists that some types of cancer may not be caused by viruses.

Some researchers believe cancer can eventually be prevented through control of the body's immune system. Scientists at the Institute for Cancer Research in Philadelphia are trying to find out how certain chemicals, viruses, X rays, and advancing age apparently weaken or suppress the body's immunologic defenses, allowing cancer to develop. Investigators at the Tumor Biology Laboratory of the University of Florida hope to develop tests to measure the body's immune response, and to learn why some persons reject cancer and others are susceptible to it.

Molecular biologists are looking into a more futuristic possibility—genetic engineering. During the last decade, biologists have learned a great deal about how cells function. Cancer, regardless of its causes, is a derangement of this function. By altering the molecular events in a cancer cell, it might be possible to change the cell back to normal. Such an approach could work even if vaccines fail, or if viruses do not turn out to be an important cause of cancer.

Similarly, if "turned on" C-type particles cause malignancy, it could be possible to "turn off" the particles. This possibly could take the form of injections to prevent cancer.

Although no one knows which of these approaches will eventually succeed, scientists are highly optimistic about the future.

EATING OURSELVES TO DEATH [7]

The buttons on Terry Benbow's gray-striped vest strain to contain a fullness befitting a man who can afford to eat anything he wants and often does. Each workday he packs

[7] From "Our Daily Bread," by Mary Bralove, staff reporter. *Wall Street Journal.* p 1. Ja. 6, '71. Reprinted by permission.

away a hearty breakfast, lunches with clients at a private Wall Street club and then, if business meetings don't delay him, hops a Staten Island ferry home to an ample dinner with his family.

That dinner typically consists of a healthy slab of meat —a good cut of roast beef, perhaps, or a steak—accompanied by potatoes or rice, vegetables, salad and dessert. There's no bemoaning "meat loaf again" at the Terence Benbow household. Mr. Benbow, a partner in a Wall Street law firm, makes enough money that his wife doesn't have to concern herself with food budgets. When Gloria Benbow shops, she can pass up the supermarket specials and pick her pleasure from the 8,000 or so other items to be found on the grocery shelves.

But does the fact that the Benbows can afford to eat well mean that they eat wisely? Not necessarily. Increasingly, nutritionists and doctors worry that millions of middle-class and upper-middle-class Americans like the Benbows are overfed and undernourished.

To support their contentions, the doctors cite some surprising facts. A 1965-66 Department of Agriculture survey reported that "poor diets were found at higher income levels, even the highest." In a review of studies of vitamin and mineral nutrition from 1950 to 1968 among Americans above poverty status, doctors found that "the nutrition of a significant proportion of the American public is inadequate and has become worse during the past ten years."

Nutritionists estimate that 10 per cent of the U.S. population is anemic while, paradoxically, 25 per cent of Americans are seriously overweight—a condition that can lead to early death from heart, circulatory, kidney or other diseases. By age forty, most American men have an excess of cholesterol in their bloodstreams that doctors suspect is a major cause of "premature" heart attacks. Of the 600,000 deaths attributed to heart disease every year, 165,000 fall into the premature category because they involve persons under sixty-five.

Dietary habits may be at least partly responsible, nutritionists suspect, for a variety of common health complaints ranging from hypertension (too much salt on your food) to irritability, insomnia and anxiety (all attributable in some cases to vitamin shortages). Doctors blame self-inflicted malnutrition—usually as a result of unnecessary and unsupervised dieting—for chronic deficiencies of calcium, vitamins A and C and iron among many teen-age girls, and they say that failure to eat properly often lies behind many of the health complaints of the elderly.

Led and Pushed

For the poor, of course, nutrition difficulties usually are caused by the lack of money to buy proper food. But that's clearly not the case with most Americans. "In the middle-income group, there's a huge amount of food available, tremendous variety and money to buy it, and all of our social customs leading us, pushing us into eating," observes Dr. Louise Mojonnier, coordinator of the Coronary Prevention Evaluation Program at the Chicago Health Research Foundation.

The problem is that through ignorance, apathy or confusion many people got led or pushed into eating the wrong things, medical experts say. Most people seem to have only a vague understanding of their nutritional needs and the values provided by various foods—and they don't get much help from the medical profession. "Often doctors are trained (in nutrition) by doctors who heard it from another doctor who made it up," says Dr. Julian B. Schorr of the New York Blood Center.

The confusion has been compounded in recent years by a flood of new foods or new variations on old foods poured onto the market by food companies, usually accompanied by hard-sell advertising campaigns that rarely impart much nutritional information.

The flood of new food products has left even nutritionists bewildered. There are "coffee creamers" that contain no milk or cream, dried "beef stroganoffs" that contain no meat and a plethora of snack products whose nutritional values—if any—are uncertain. To find out just what they're eating themselves, many nutritionists report, they often have to write the manufacturer.

Add to all this the quirks of individual taste and the hectic pace of work, school and social activities maintained by many young families, and the result is apt to be a set of haphazard eating habits that bear little relationship to nutritional needs.

The extent to which the pace of an active household affects eating habits is obvious at the Benbow home on New York's Staten Island. Besides Mr. and Mrs. Benbow, the family consists of two teen-age sons and a daughter who entered the University of Michigan this fall as a freshman. Along with being a housewife and mother, Mrs. Benbow is a part-time teacher of history and English and an accomplished singer who regularly appears as a soloist in a local Episcopal church.

The family members begin to go their own dietary ways first thing in the morning. The boys—sixteen-year-old Christopher and fourteen-year-old Jonathan—arise about 7:30 ("They'd rather sleep than eat," says their mother) and grab a quick, light, breakfast such as tea and muffin or an "instant breakfast" concoction before heading off to school. "I gulp it out the door," says Jon.

Mr. Benbow gets up about 8:20 to a full breakfast of eggs, toast, coffee and juice. His wife usually skips breakfast, she says, settling for a cup of coffee after she drives him to the ferry.

The boys eat lunch at school, Mr. Benbow eats in Manhattan, and Mrs. Benbow, at home, eats lightly if at all. Two or three nights a week, dinner is served in two shifts because Mr. Benbow is held up by a late meeting at work.

Even on weekends, the family has so many activities that meals rarely are eaten together. "The one time we all sat down to three meals a day together was the three weeks we spent on Cape Cod" ... says Mrs. Benbow.

One result is that different members of the family have widely different eating habits. Mr. Benbow is a three-squares-a-day man, but stops there. "I'm not a snacker or a cruncher," he says. The boys, on the other hand, eat less at mealtimes but make up for it in the evening with several cans of soda pop and snacks of potato chips, popcorn and pretzels. "We wait until 7:30, until the good TV shows are on, and then we get food in front of the boob-tube," says Jon.

Mrs. Benbow figures she is about fifteen pounds over-weight, and, she says, "I'm perpetually on a diet, like most housewives." Her husband, who is five feet, eight inches tall, weighs around 175 pounds, well over the range of 137 to 151 most medical charts recommend for his height. "Perhaps I should worry about it, but I don't," he says. "I've been chubby all my life, and I've learned to live with it."

Medical experts do worry about excess weight, however. Some consider obesity to be a far more serious problem among middle-class Americans than vitamin shortages and the like. "Nutrition is killing us," declares Dr. Grant Gwin-up, director of the Metabolic Research Laboratory at the University of California. "We ought to be focusing not on the baloney of did you get your vitamins but, 'Look at you, Mr. America, you're fat and you're dying.' That guy with a paunch would live five years longer if he would keep lean." ...

Many nutritionists simply hedge on the question of an appropriate diet, suggesting that people should eat a little bit of everything and not too much of any one thing. But most agree on at least a few basic suggestions.

Cut Down on Sweets

First of all, they urge that Americans should cut dow
on the amount of sweet goods consumed—candy, cake, pastr
and the like. They also urge that housewives start servin;
more green vegetables such as broccoli, spinach and othe
leafy greens, which are rich in the vitamins and iron man
people chronically lack.

(Women of all ages are particularly likely to be shor
of iron. At study of 114 college women found stored iror
absent in two thirds. According to a food executive, anothe
study of college women revealed iron shortages in all bu
one. Researchers discovered she ate hamburgers and spaghett
just as everyone else did—but she cooked in a corroding
iron pot. Nutritionists hasten to add, though, that no on(
has proved iron from a pot can be absorbed and used b)
the body.)

Nutritionists warn against overcooking vegetables, whicl
can destroy many of the natural vitamins. On the othe
hand, they note that some vegetables—carrots, for example
—are more nutritious when cooked than when eaten raw

There's a need for people to reconsider some of thei
old ideas and eating habits, many food experts say. There'
no reason, for instance, a person can't eat a cheese sand-
wich, a hamburger or even strawberry shortcake with milk
for breakfast and still be as well off nutritionally as if he
had a more traditional menu, nutritionists point out.

A Good Word for Hamburger

A common food fallacy is the belief that steak is
uniquely rich in protein; nutritionists say hamburger is
just as good. Nutritionists say, moreover, that protein-rich
vegetables or grains—like wheat, rice or beans—often can
and should be substituted for high-cholesterol animal
meats.

Such a change is in line with the recent recommendation
of a Federal heart-study panel that Americans cut down their

onsumption of all types of saturated fats. (For laymen's pur-
oses, saturated fats are usually defined as those that are solid
t room temperature.) Among the foods that should be
voided, the panel said, are egg yolks, butter fat (found in
milk, butter and certain types of cheese), fatty meats, shell-
ish and fat-rich baked goods and candies. Whenever pos-
ible, foods should be prepared with vegetable oils, which
re unsaturated and usually far lower in cholesterol.

Though the panel acknowledged that firm evidence link-
ng dietary fats and cholesterol to heart disease still is lack-
ng, it argued that medical suspicion of such a link is great
nough to warrant changes in dietary habits.

Nation of Nibblers

While some nutritionists are trying to change Americans'
ating habits, others feel it's up to the food companies to
nake their products more healthful and adapt to the existing
abits of a "nation of nibblers." Jean Mayer, professor of
nutrition at Harvard University's School of Public Health,
ays he feels it's "too late in the day" to try to get Americans
o stop eating snacks. He and others recommend that food
companies add nutriments to the products people insist on
ating.

Many food products, of course, have long been enriched
with extra vitamins and minerals—notably bread, flour and
milk. But now food companies are slowly responding to the
idea of enriching other products as well. Nabisco, for example, has added some vitamins to its cookie and cracker
products.

Food producers point out, however, that it's possible to
get too many vitamins. Some, such as vitamins A and D, can
be toxic when taken in extremely large doses—more than
thirty times the normal requirements. Too much vitamin A
can lead to loss of hair, drying of the skin, and bone and
joint pain, while vitamin D overdoses may result in nausea,
diarrhea and weight loss.

But experts figure it would take something like a nutri
tional panic for people to devour such overdoses. Far mor
worrisome, most nutritionists contend, is the problem simpl
of getting enough nutriments into Americans.

THE "HEADACHE HUNTERS" MEET
THE ANXIOUS AMERICAN [8]

At night, while she slept, her right hand turned an
reached out in an agonized twist. In the day, her hours wer
filled with the nightmare of constant headache—"blurre
vision, the feeling of constant pressure in the head." In th
evening, she had hallucinations—"ugly faces and whispering
I tried to scream, but I couldn't."

She had her own diagnosis: "I was afraid I was going
bananas."

Now she sat in an examination room in a private head
ache clinic in Chicago. She had her "sample book" with her
She was an artist of extraordinary talent. Once she'd spent he
days, in her suburban home, on this art. But not since th
headaches began: "I couldn't concentrate well enough."
Months without her art. Months of torment for herself and
her husband. And now it was over. The hand was relaxed
The hallucinations were gone. And the headaches were over.

"I started sketching again last week," she said.

This young woman is one of scores of people who come
every week to the second-floor clinic in a modern building
on the north side of Chicago. They come from every walk of
life—the well-dressed, dignified lady from the suburbs, the
crew-cut physical education teacher with bleary eyes and a
running nose, the conscientious housewife from a small town
in Indiana.

They all have one thing in common: terrible, recurring
headaches. For most, the headaches are so intense and so fre-

[8] From article by freelance writer William Barry Furlong. Today's Health.
49:20-3+. Mr. '71. Today's Health is copyrighted and published by the American Medical Association.

...ent that they virtually incapacitate the victim. For a few, ...e fear is as great as the pain: "Are you sure there's nothing ...owing in there, Doctor?" asked a fearful bank teller.

"We get only the toughest cases," says Dr. Seymour Dia-...ond, codirector of the clinic and a leading researcher into ...e headache phenomenon. "If it was an uncomplicated case, ...me doctor in general practice would handle it."

The number of tough cases is going up and up. It's esti-...ated that as many as 42 million Americans experience ...vere headaches. Some 10 million of them suffer migraine ...eadaches. Millions more suffer headaches that derive from ...nsions, anxieties, or depression—headaches which interfere ...ith the way they live.

The anxious state of the American psyche—of which head-...ches are a conspicuous symptom—was reflected in an annual ...port released by the United States Public Health Service ...te in 1970: Some 5.2 million adults had suffered a nervous ...reakdown and 14.2 million adults were considered near one.

In the past, the persistence of chronic headache usually ...as regarded less as a disease than a defect. It was looked ...pon as an emotional problem, not a physical one. Indeed, ...: was thought to be the emotional reaction to anxieties. Few ...octors cared to devote tedious effort to curing the headache. ...ne woman recalls that she'd been plagued by headaches for ...wenty-four years and was told by one physician that "it was ...ll in my imagination." Another woman was told her head-...ches were the result of a negative attitude toward life.

In the last several years, headaches have been the subject ...f a great deal of enterprising research all over the world. ...ome of it took place in an atmosphere of basic research, such ...s that under Dr. Donald J. Dalessio at the Scripps Clinic in ...a Jolla, California, and that of Dr. John R. Graham at the ...leadache Research Foundation of Boston's Faulkner Hos-...ital. Some of the studies took place in an atmosphere of ...laily practice, such as at the headache clinic in Chicago and ...he Headache Unit under Dr. Arnold Friedman at Montefiore Hospital and Medical Center in New York City. Son research took place overseas, such as that by Dr. James V Lance of the University of New South Wales in Australia

The conclusion of most investigators is that there is a wa to treat headaches that will reduce the pain and allow th patient to function normally.

There is no cure-all for migraine or any kind of headach —nor is there a single cause. Physicians have found many p: tients who simultaneously display symptoms of two or mo different kinds of headache. But headache pain can be r duced or altogether eliminated with the proper treatment.

Recently, a successful businessman in his fifties came t the clinic operated by Doctor Diamond and Dr. Bernard Baltes. The patient complained of an unbearable series c headaches. That he was successful might be considered symptom: Migraine sufferers tend to be meticulous, har driving types who try to push themselves to extreme leve of accomplishment. They have included such diverse person alities as Thomas Jefferson, Sigmund Freud, Lew Alcind (the altitudinous basketball player), and writer Lewis Ca roll (whose *Alice in Wonderland* might have been inspire in part, from hallucinatory migraine).

But this businessman had not suffered any such hea aches before age fifty—"and migraine tends to decrease as ag goes up," says Doctor Diamond. So Doctors Diamond an Baltes simply let the patient talk. "So often it's just a matte of letting an individual 'ventilate' his problems," says Do tor Diamond.

But this particular patient seemed to have no problems at least none that were causing him any perceptible turmoi He displayed no signs of organic disease, showed no represse emotions, no simmering hostilities. He was satisfied with life In short, he was disturbingly well-adjusted.

And then one day it all came out: He was the victim o the "soy sauce syndrome."

The man talked enthusiastically of his fondness for Chi-
ese food; he'd dine at a Chinese restaurant at least once a
eek. Doctor Diamond remembered that some persons ex-
erience a toxic reaction to the monosodium glutamate in
oy sauce. The reaction causes a dilation of the blood vessels
round the brain. That vascular swelling is similar to the
echanism of a migraine headache. The patient was suffer-
ig every symptom of a migraine, but not because of a
igraine.

Doctor Diamond urged that the man give up Chinese
ood—or a least the soy sauce on the side. The headaches
ased immediately.

Toxic reactions and allergies are among the more subtle
auses of headaches, though these factors may be difficult to
etect. . . .

According to Doctor Diamond, many people use physical
roblems as a shield against their emotional ones. It is not
urposeful; it is almost reflexive—the patient's body "sends
essages which he himself does not completely understand."

Some cannot be treated successfully. Doctor Diamond
emembers an attractive, well-to-do woman who accepted
reatment right up to the point where it seemed she might
e substantially relieved of headache pain. Then she gave up
reatment. The reason: Her headaches were a protective re-
ction against her husband, who was unfaithful. The wife
sed the headache as a shield against him, perhaps as a device
o win sympathy from others, possibly to inspire guilt in her
usband.

The research of the last few years has led to slightly dif-
erent classification of headaches. A grouping developed for
he American Association for the Study of Headaches has
welve classifications which fit generally into three broad
ategories: the "vascular" headache, the "muscle contrac-
ion" headache (akin to the pain felt in the muscle area
where the neck joins the head), and the "traction" or organ-
cally caused headache.

The first step in treating a headache, therefore, is to dete mine whether it is being caused by a specific illness. . . .

Clinical experience suggests that the chemical factor pla an important role in headaches. For example, headache pai frequently accompanies menstrual changes in a woman.

Research has explored not only the chemistry but th mechanism of migraine, as well as the kind of person mo likely to suffer this kind of headache. It is known now, fo instance, that the migraine sufferer is more likely to be woman than a man and that, as a general rule, she is likel to be trim, neatly dressed, intelligent, with an inclination t speak quickly, and with a body cycle that involves a mornin lassitude followed by an evening peak. The man who suffe from migraine is likely to be ambitious, with an exaggerate sense of responsibility, a perfectionist towards himself an others.

The typical migraine sufferer has a family history of heac aches. She also has a tendency to worry, to possess rigid stanc ards, to exhibit a strong need for approval, to be sensitive t criticism, to feel a sense of frustration about life. Often th migraine victim is enduring a suppressed rage or hostility t certain factors or persons in her life.

Doctor Diamond notes that many migraine victims di play the "first-child" syndrome. That is, as firstborns, the feel some inner responsibility to be active and accomplishin

"Headache patients tend to build lives with too many e vironmental demands," says Doctor Diamond. "They are e tremely sensitive to this overload." One result is that th continuing pressures within their own lives touch off th migraine.

"Often the problems of life are not the inner conflicts c a person but the defenses set up against them," he says. . . .

"Muscle contraction" headaches . . . commonly calle "tension" headaches . . . are [usually] recognized by a tau ness in the muscles, usually at the back of the neck. This typ is frequently a response to a stress-producing situation an can be treated—by the patient himself—with aspirin or othe pain-killers. Of course, the headaches may recur because the tension continues at a high level. Frequently, this is a continuing response to the personality of the patient.

The typical victim is the sort of person who tends to work too hard, relax too little, and be overly concerned about his or her ability to perform a task or cope with a situation [notes Doctor Friedman of Montefiore Hospital]. An individual may feel threatened by the demands of a job or profession, and sometimes those fears may be unrealistic, although understandable.

He recalls one capable young attorney who dreaded to make court appearances. It was not that he feared failure or was incompetent; even his critics considered his performance consistently superior. But he developed a high degree of tension because he expected unfailing excellence of himself.

"As he learned to expect a little less of himself"—and to recognize each situation demands, and inspires, different levels of performance in a man—"the headaches gradually became fewer, finally vanishing," reports Doctor Friedman.

In this case, the tension was caused by anxiety, uncomplicated by other factors.

Where anxiety alone is present—even a persistent anxiety—the patient can be treated, usually by use of tranquilizers. When used carefully under a doctor's care, tranquilizers may relieve headache and the anxiety that caused it (even though the patient might continue to encounter stress-filled situations).

Antiheadache drugs not only work against the chemical changes which cause headaches in the depressed person, but they work against the depression itself. Thus they attack both the symptom—the headache—and its cause.

But it is not always obvious that depression is the cause of a chronic headache. The patient may not know he is depressed. He's been feeling this way so long that it seems like his natural state of being. Depression, Doctor Diamond points out, is an enduring condition in certain persons. "It might last anywhere from a few months in a young person to six to eight years in an older one," he says. Thus the depression becomes so constant that it seems "normal" behavior to the patient and his family. They may not identify depression as a factor; the doctor must discern it through his own examination.

Even greater difficulty is encountered when several factors are present in the cause of chronic headache. For example, a depressed person might also be suffering from anxiety. But he should be given treatment for one or the other quite carefully—a tranquilizer given a deeply depressed person might throw him into a deeper depression. So the physician usually will work on one aspect of the headache problem and, when it is under control, go on to the next.

Perhaps the most serious problem comes when both vascular and muscle-contraction headaches are present at the same time—say, a migraine attack combined with a depression-induced headache.

"Just worrying about getting a headache can deepen a depression which may itself cause a depression headache," suggests Doctor Baltes.

The migraine so possesses its victims that often he or she worries about getting one from his first waking moment; the worry then induces a headache, which confirms his fears —and helps start his worry again.

Such a patient offers a baffling series of headache symptoms—nothing so simple as a migraine (which takes place in one part of the head) or the tautness of neck muscle (as in a muscle contraction). His pain appears in different places at different times with different intensities for different durations. The patient, of course, does not know the difference between the headaches, so he cannot sort out the symptoms. The doctor must search carefully by talking to the individual.

Successful attacks on a combination of headaches can be made with thoughtful diagnosis and treatment.

Thus there is hope for relief of pain for victims of persistent headaches. Yet these successes in treating headaches are only a start on what some day might be accom-

)lished for those unfortunate refugees, forever on the run
rom a pain they feared they could never escape.

STRESS IN OUR LIVES [9]

Conditions of stress face us no matter which way we
urn. War, crime, revolt of youth, drug use, sex problems,
:rowding, crises at home and at work—all these things pro-
luce tension, frustration and harassment at a level that often
ipproaches the threshold of toleration. W. H. Auden calls
•ur era the age of anxiety. Others use labels like rat race
nd the "stoned age" to describe our society and these times.
Γhe average citizen's hopes for a serene life are blasted time
nd again. Cherished values are battered, religious leaders
;ive currency to Nietzsche's notion that God is dead, com-
)uters depersonalize many of life's interchanges, and doctors
;enerate moral complexities by prolonging life artificially
nd transplanting human organs. Alienation increases and
he problems of attaining peace, justice, orderly change and
ι clean environment grow more complex.

Stress, however, is not all bad. If not excessive, it can
erve a useful purpose, such as preparing an individual to
neet a threat or fulfilling his need for adventure. Even ex-
reme stress can be constructive if it enables an individual
o act effectively for survival. Samuel Silverman, a psy-
hiatrist, contends that stress is not only useful but neces-
ary. "A certain amount of stimulation and excitation—of
he right kind and under the right conditions—appears to
»e necessary for the maintenance of a healthy 'psychophy-
ical tone.'" Stress stimulates physical and mental work,
ιelping the person challenge difficult problems.

Stress is thought to be needed even for the ordinary plea-
ures of living. Dr. Harry J. Johnson, a prominent mental

⁹ From "Stress in Modern Life," by William Gerber, staff writer. *Editorial
'.esearch Reports.* 2 no 3:529-30, 539-42. Jl. 15, '70. Reprinted by permission.
•r. Gerber, an educator and consultant, is the author of several books and a
)ntributor to American and British periodicals.

hygienist, contends that "Life without stress is like sou
without salt." Moreover, the physiological side effects o
pleasurable stress need not be harmful. Dr. Hans Selye, a
professor of psychology at McGill University, wrote tha
"A game of tennis or even a passionate kiss can produc
considerable stress without conspicuous damage." Chicag
psychoanalyst Karen Horney has explored the shadow are
between good and harmful stress. "Riding a roller-coaste
with some apprehension may make it more thrilling," sh
observed, "whereas doing it with strong anxiety will mak
it a torture." The achievement in our lives of a beneficia
and not excessive exposure to stress requires a deeper knowl
edge than most people have of themselves and the challenge
they face. It requires a knowledge of the causes and effect
of stress, of the machinery by which the body and min
attempt to cope with stress, and of controls and outlets. . .

Alvin Toffler, of the Russell Sage Foundation [and autho
of *Future Shock*], fears that "We are creating an environmen
so filled with astonishments, twists, reversals, eruption
mind-jangling crises, and innovations as to test the limit
of man's adaptive capacity."—"We are setting the stage fo
future shock on a vast scale." ["Future Shock," by Alvi
Toffler. *Horizon*. p 82. Spring '70. Article adapted fron
his book, published by Random House, 1970.] Some psychol
ogists and social scientists believe that stress in social rela
tions could be eased by decreasing the size of institution
communities and governments. There are others who believ
that tighter law enforcement would promote the order an
security needed for a relaxation of anxieties in urban Ame
ica. Still others maintain that if the government provide
more help to the less privileged it would reduce stress cause
by deprivation or discrimination.

Some young people have rejected material success as
primary goal in life. They tend to "hang loose" in a job an
face stress with equanimity. Other youths reject the earnin
of money through a regular job because they consider tha

way of living to be cursed with the stress of competitiveness. Young people, with renewable wellsprings of energy, may be better equipped to cope with stress than their elders. If the young are idealistic and channel their energy in efforts to improve society, two kinds of benefits may result. First, such labors are wholesome for the individual himself, and they may also enable sympathizers who do not march or carry a sign to let off steam vicariously. Second, these efforts may have a useful social effect in alerting the public to an area in need of attention. Moreover, doing volunteer work for a good cause may lessen the feeling of entrapment and powerlessness and add to the individual's sense of belonging.

"To get physically tired," heart specialist Paul Dudley White said, "is the best antidote for nervous tension." Play tennis, chop wood, punch a bag—any number of fatiguing activities are good for releasing belligerent impulses aroused by the stress of living. Yelling at the umpire or even watching a violence-filled movie may also provide outlets for aggressive impulses. Aristotle said that attending a tragic drama purges the soul of its tensions by arousing and then exhausting pity and fear.

Building Up Resilience Through Ego Strength

Seeking an unrelated outlet for one's frustrations is not always the best therapy, however. It may be beneficial for the person to acknowledge the stresses that afflict him and try to work around them. Erik Erikson [professor of human development and lecturer in psychiatry at Harvard University] contends that we should confront our anxieties. The first step is "to train our fear . . . to remain an accurate measure and warning of that which man must fear." Terence Moore, psychologist of London's Child Guidance Training Center, wrote:

This quality of resilience apparently varies from birth, and very probably has a genetic component; but it seems likely, too, that it may be fostered or reduced by environmental conditions, especially in the early years. Adults can sometimes show children how to cope successfully with everyday stresses. Or lacking understanding or sympathy, they can very easily undermine the child's efforts and increase the stress to the breaking point, when tears or a tantrum will result.

Resilience depends partly on ego strength, or self-esteem. Psychologists and social workers in recent years have developed a technique for bolstering the ego resources of persons undergoing severe stress. This technique, called crisis intervention, is applied especially to people who appear to be heading for a breakdown because of bereavement, fear of surgery, or other identifiable causes. Visits by close friends, reassurance, encouragement, praise, explanations, and opportunities for a good cry are parts of the technique.

Crisis intervention to promote resilience in periods of stress has been tried also in cases of social turmoil. During the time of riots that tore many other American cities in 1968, Mayor John V. Lindsay made himself visible in ghetto areas of New York, offering needed support that encouraged people to mourn instead of riot. In Boston, at the request of Mayor Kevin White, soul-singer James Brown stayed on television to serve as a calming influence. Brown also appeared later on radio and television in Washington for the same purpose.

Finding a Balance Between Ambition and Repose

A complete absence of stress is not an admirable ideal. As Hans Selye noted in *The Stress of Life* (1956): "Comfort and security make it easier for us to enjoy the good things in life, but they are not, in themselves, great and enjoyable aims." Even as a temporary measure for therapeutic purposes, the absence of stress is not necessarily a wise goal. Selye wrote: "I have always been against the advice of physicians who would send a high-strung, extremely active business executive to a long, enforced exile in some health resort, with a view of relieving him from stress by absolute inactivity."

A balance between ambition and repose would seem to be desirable, but there are exceptions. Eugene E. Levitt, a professor of clinical psychology, said: "We can only wonder vainly what De Quincey or Poe or Van Gogh would have produced if they had been emotionally better balanced." Selye's suggestion is that one should "live and express his personality at a tempo and in a manner best suited to his inherited talents, under the prevailing social conditions."

One key to achieving a proper balance is the principle of variety. Dr. Johnson offers these suggestions for applying that principle:

Every desk-bound worker should leave his chair at least once every two hours and walk about his office for a few minutes.

Chairmen should call for occasional ten-minute intermissions during meetings, breaking up both tension and boredom.

Relaxation does not mean rest; it means a change of scene, a change of activity.

The best cure for tension fatigue is walking.

In the Old Testament wisdom of Ecclesiastes, there is a proper season for everything. Thus we should allow a time for ambition and a time for repose. Modern medicine holds that the division between stress and relaxation should apply not only to daily matters but to life as a whole. Plans such as these, unfortunately, have a way of being exploded by stressful events that were not anticipated. Therefore, the individual needs to build two things: a plan for balance between stress and nonstress, and sufficient ego strength to endure the destruction of the plan.

THE CONSEQUENCES OF MEDICAL ADVANCES [10]

With its mixture of science and social service, medicine is particularly sensitive to the social scene and, conversely, new developments in medicine affect society. Science increases understanding of biological and medical problems. How this understanding is applied, however, is society's concern and new developments in medicine pose real problems for all of us today. . . .

[I wish to] discuss two related problems which are already upon us.

The first concerns the cost-benefit of extending life as the goal of medicine. Most physicians, I believe, would qualify this goal by inserting some statement regarding the quality of the life that is being extended but this already involves the physician in value judgments which society has not delegated to him to make.

Medical science allows us to prolong the lives of patients suffering from renal [kidney] failure. Experts have estimated for the Bureau of the Budget that the expected costs of adding nine years to the patient's life by hemodialysis would be $71,000; adding seventeen years by kidney transplantation would cost $44,500. The difficulties in estimating survival rates and dollar costs limit the accuracy of these estimates. But with costs of this magnitude several questions arise.

Most patients can't bear the cost of such treatment: $5,000 to $14,000 per year for dialysis, $13,000 for a kidney transplant. Should the Government underwrite these costs? Using these estimates, experts have concluded that the first six years, ending in 1975, of a national program designed to provide dialysis for about 18,000 patients and transplants for more than 4,000 patients would cost $800 million to

[10] From "Social Consequences of New Developments in Medicine," by Alexander Leaf, M.D., Jackson Professor of Clinical Medicine, Harvard University. *Bulletin of the Atomic Scientists.* 26:21-2. Ja. '70. Reprinted by permission of Science and Public Affairs, the *Bulletin of the Atomic Scientists.* Copyright © 1970 by the Educational Foundation for Nuclear Science.

$1 billion. One may argue that the dollar costs are not unreasonable for the lives involved. But if our resources are limited—and at some point they must be—we must consider the costs of diverting these dollars from other uses.

But dollars are not the only resource which is limited. The technically skilled, the physicians and nurses as well as hospitals are not available for such a mass activity. The pool of these resources is far from sufficient to man a mass program at this time and still minister to the other health needs of our nation. In fact, it is not unlikely that such a venture might inhibit further acquisition of understanding of kidney disease and thus postpone the day when effective preventative measures can be taken to avoid the need for dialysis and transplant.

If resources are limited we should compare the costs of a dialysis and kidney transplant program with that of other health needs. It is estimated that early detection of cancer of the cervix through "Pap" tests might save 9,000 lives a year. Prevention of blindness from glaucoma by early detection and treatment, or a preventative dental health program, are examples of programs which would not be life saving but which would enhance the quality of life and the well-being of thousands or millions. The task of allocating resources arises everywhere. With the national expenditures for health annually already in excess of $50 billion, careful planning is very much in order.

Recently the General Executive Committee of the Massachusetts General Hospital considered the advisability of commencing heart transplants at our hospital. With a cardiac surgery team that we think is unexcelled anywhere and with considerable experience in kidney transplants and the immunologic problems involved in organ compatibility, it seemed to many of the staff that this was the logical place for such innovations to take place. However, sober thinking made us ask a number of pertinent questions. Should we be embarking on programs which tie up large numbers of our staff for the care of a single patient? On the national health scene there is an absolute shortage of physicians to care for society's needs. Nurses have been in such short supply that many hospitals in the last couple of years have had to reduce their bed occupancy because of the nursing shortage at a time when our hospital beds are oversubscribed. One heart transplant case can be expected to tie up four or five nurses for a six-to-twelve week period, whereas elsewhere in the hospital the same number of nurses might minister to the needs of twenty or more patients.

By embarking on this kind of surgery would we be contributing to the mistaken view, which some segments of the public hold, that this is a therapeutic procedure rather than a research project? Would we hasten our knowledge of the immunological problems involved by adding heart transplants to the other organs we are transplanting when the immunological reactions in these other organs are the limiting factor in the success of the transplantation? Will the considerable costs and medical resources committed to heart transplant restrict the research that is needed into the basic causes of arteriosclerosis and coronary heart disease? What about the health needs of several thousand normal children which could be looked after for the cost of one heart transplant? How do we equate their health and well-being with the life of one oldster? These are no longer questions which the cardiac surgeon alone can answer, nor a single department. One member of the General Executive Committee alleged that such deliberations constituted an infringement on the rights of each surgeon and department to decide what therapeutic measures will or will not be offered to the sick. But we are now faced with decisions which don't affect the personnel or resources of a single department. How we decide will foreclose other options for the entire hospital.

In general terms one may summarize a major social

problem affecting medicine as that of establishing priorities
for what medicine shall treat and what it shall not treat.
Science has provided understanding and technology has
provided means for helping care for our ill and aged. At
the same time costs for such intensive, personnel-consuming
efforts have increased to exorbitant proportions. The individual, aside from exceptional instances, cannot bear the
cost of such treatment. Society, more specifically government, must underwrite costs. This produces the para-
doxical situation of public funds being used to insure the
welfare of fewer individuals whose survival requires increasingly costly services. When resources are limited, who
decides which members of society will benefit from popular
support and which, if need be, will be cut off from support? The more we waste our resources on futile and worth-
less military expenditures the sooner we reach the limit
of resources which can be made available for the nation's
health needs.

Defining Death

Another social problem arising from recent improvements in medical technology has to do with the definition
of death. Legally, death is defined as occurring when the
heart stops beating. Today, with assisted respiratory devices and heart pacing, it is possible to keep a patient
breathing and his heart beating for long, perhaps indefinite,
periods of time. This has proved invaluable in tiding
patients over potentially fatal periods of respiratory or
cardiac arrest. But what happens when these assisting devices
are used in a patient who unfortunately has undergone
irreparable brain damage? Is the patient still alive because his heart is beating even though the cells in his brain
are dead and show no evidence of activity on an electro-
encephalogram? This is the legal status of such an unfortunate individual. The physician has not the right or permission to shut off the assisting devices and allow the heart

to stop beating so the patient may be pronounced dead, even when the possibility of recovery of brain function is nil. The possibility exists that such an action may result in murder charges being pressed against the physician. Clearly a society which is unable to distinguish whether its members are dead or alive may expect difficulties thereby.

Organ Transplants

One difficulty which has already arisen relates to pressures from another development in medicine—transplantation of organs. Patients who die serve as donors for transplant of various organs. But if cadaveric organs are to be used for transplantation, the shorter the period of anoxia [absence of oxygen] to which they have been subjected, the less likely they are to suffer damage before transplantation, and the more likely is the transplantation to be a success. Thus it is advantageous to the surgeon to be able to remove organs from a subject who can be pronounced "dead" even while his heart is still beating and perfusion of the donor organs is maintained. The ability to keep patients alive by life-assisting devices and the need for donor organs for transplantation leads to a public concept of a conflict of interest among physicians. . . .

In summary, the increased understanding of medical problems resulting from scientific investigation may, as with understanding of nature in any field, be used for socially desirable or undesirable ends. Society must decide on the applications of this understanding. Even with desirable medical applications to be supported, society must make some difficult moral judgments which will indicate whether these new technological advances in medicine are applied to the benefit of all or to just a few of its members.

BIBLIOGRAPHY

An asterisk (*) preceding a reference indicates that the article or a part of it has been reprinted in this book.

BOOKS, PAMPHLETS, AND DOCUMENTS

Andersen, R. and Anderson, O. W. A decade of health services. University of Chicago Press. '68.

Anderson, O. W. Voluntary health insurance in two cities: a survey of subscriber households [by the author and the staff of the National Opinion Research Center, University of Chicago]. Harvard University Press. '57.

Atchley, D. W. Physician, healer and scientist. Macmillan. '61.

Augenstein, L. G. Come let us play God. Harper. '69.

Babbie, E. R. Science and morality in medicine: a survey of medical educators. University of California Press. '70.

Balint, Michael, ed. A study of doctors. Tavistock Publications. '66.

*Block, Irvin. The health of the poor. (Pamphlet no 435) Public Affairs Committee, Inc. 381 Park Ave. S. New York 10016. '69.

Bowers, J. Z. ed. Medical schools for the modern world. Johns Hopkins Press. '70.

Brahdy, Leopold, ed. Diease and injury. Lippincott. '61.

Bruess, C. E. and Fisher, J. T. Selected readings in health. Macmillan. '70.

Carnegie Commission on the Future of Higher Education. Higher education and the nation's health: policies for medical and dental education; a special report and recommendations. McGraw. '70.

Chandler, C. A. Famous modern men of medicine. Dodd. '65.

Ciba Foundation. Ethics in medical progress; with special reference to transplantation; ed. by G. E. W. Wolstenholme and Maeve O'Connor. Little. '66.

Clark, D. W. and MacMahon, B. W. Preventive medicine. Little. '67.

Comfort, Alex. The anxiety makers. Dell. '70.

Cope, Oliver. Man, mind and medicine: the doctor's education. Lippincott. '68.

Cope, Oliver and Zacharias, Jerrold. Medical education reconsidered. Lippincott. '66.

Corcoran, A. C. ed. A mirror up to medicine. Lippincott. '61.

Cray, Ed. In failing health; the medical crisis and the A.M.A. Bobbs. '71.

Crichton, Michael. Five patients: the hospital explained. Knopf. '70.
   Excerpts. Atlantic. 225:49-57. Mr. '70. High cost of cure: how a hospital bill grows 17 feet long; Ladies Home Journal. 87:34+. Jl. '70.

Cunningham, R. M. Third world of medicine. McGraw. '68.

Cutler, D. R. ed. Updating life and death. Beacon. '69.

Deitz, E. H. W. You can work in the health services; ed. by C. L. Byerly. Day. '68.

De Kruif, Paul. Men against death. Harcourt. '32.

Dubos, René. Man, medicine and environment. Praeger. '68.

Dubos, René. Mirage of health. (Anchor Books) Doubleday. '66. paper ed.

Eberle, Irmengarde. Modern medical discoveries. new rev. ed. Crowell. '68.

Edmunds, Vincent. Ethical responsibility in medicine. Williams & Wilkins. '67.

Ehrenreich, Barbara and Ehrenreich, John. The American health empire: power, profits and politics. Random House. '71.

Evang, Karl. Health service, society and medicine. Oxford University Press. '60.

Evans, L. J. The crisis in medical education. University of Michigan Press. '64.

Fein, Rashi. Doctor shortage: an economic diagnosis. Brookings Institution. '67.

Fletcher, J. F. Morals and medicine. Beacon. '60.

Flexner, Abraham. Abraham Flexner: an autobiography. Simon & Schuster. '60.

Fortune, Editors of, eds. Our ailing medical system. Harper. '70.

French, R. M. The dynamics of health care. McGraw. '68.

Friedrich, Rudolph. Frontiers of medicine. Macmillan. '64.

Galdston, Iago. Medicine in transition. University of Chicago Press. '65.

Gelfand, Michael. Philosophy and ethics in medicine. Williams & Wilkins. '68.

Grant, J. B. Health care for the community. Johns Hopkins Press. '63.

Gregg, Alan. Challenges to contemporary medicine. Columbia University Press. '56.

Gross, Martin. The doctors: an analysis of the American physician. Random House. '66.

Heller, J. H. Of mice, men, and molecules. Scribner. '60.

Hobson, William. World health and history. Williams & Wilkins. '63.

Horowitz, Milton. Educating tomorrow's doctors. Appleton. '64.

Inglis, Brian. The case for unorthodox medicine. Putnam. '65.

Johnson, H. J. Eat, drink, be merry, and live longer. Doubleday. '68.

Kiev, Ari. Magic, faith and healing. Free Press. '64.

Klarman, H. E. The economics of health. Columbia University Press. '65.

Klarman, H. E. ed. Empirical studies in health economics. Johns Hopkins Press. '70.

Knowles, J. H. ed. Hospitals, doctors and the public interest. Harvard University Press. '65.

Knowles, J. H. ed. Views of medical education and medical care. Harvard University Press. '68.

Koos, E. L. Health in Regionville: what the people thought and did about it. Hafner. '54.

Lain, E. P. Doctor and patient. McGraw. '69.

Lapage, Geoffrey. Man against disease. Abelard-Schuman. '64.

Lasagna, Louis. Life, death and the doctor. Knopf. '68.

Leach, Gerald. The biocrats. McGraw. '70.

Lieberman, D. L. ed. Pre-med: the foundation of a medical career. McGraw. '68.

Longmore, Donald. Machines in medicine. Aldus. '69.

Lush, Brandon, ed. Concepts of medicine. Pergamon. '61.

Magraw, R. M. Ferment in medicine. Saunders. '66.

Mayo, Charles. Mayo: the story of my family and my career. Doubleday. '68.

Mechanic, David. Medical sociology: a selective view. Macmillan. '68.

Mencher, Samuel. British private medical practice and the national health service. University of Pittsburgh Press. '68.

National Academy of Sciences. Reform of medical education. The Academy. 2101 Constitution Ave. N.W. Washington, D.C. 20418. '70.

Neal, H. E. Disease detectives; your career in medical research. Messner. '68.

Nourse, A. E. So you want to be a doctor. Harper. '63.

O'Malley, C. D. ed. History of medical education. University of California Press. '70.

Pappworth, M. H. Human guinea pigs. Beacon. '68.

Parran, Thomas and others. Hospitals, medical care and public responsibility. University of Pittsburgh Press. '62.

Pinckney, E. R. You can prevent illness. Collier. '62.

Poole, Lynn and Poole, Gray. Electronics in medicine. McGraw. '64.

Ramsey, Paul. The patient as person: exploration in medical ethics. Yale University Press. '70.

Rapport, S. B. and Wright, Helen, eds. Great adventures in medicine. Dial. '61.

Reynolds, F. W. and Barsam, P. C. Adult health; services for the chronically ill and aged. Macmillan. '67.

Richmond, J. B. Currents in American medicine: a developmental view of medical care and education. Harvard University Press. '69.

Rosengren, W. R. and Lefton, Mark. Hospitals and patients. Atherton. '70.

Rosinski, E. F. and Spencer, F. J. The assistant medical officer: the training of the medical auxiliary in developing countries. University of North Carolina Press. '65.

Roueché, Berton. Eleven blue men. Little. '54.

Roueché, Berton. A man named Hoffman. Little. '65.

Rutstein, D. D. Coming revolution in medicine. MIT Press. '67.

Schmeck, H. M., Jr. The semi-artificial man. Walker and Co. '65.

Serbein, O. N. Paying for medical care in the U.S. Columbia University Press. '53.

Sheps, C. G. Needed research in health and medical care. University of North Carolina Press. '54.

Somers, H. M. and Somers, A. R. Doctors, patients and health insurance. Brookings Institution. '61.

omers, H. M. and Somers, A. R. Medicare and the hospitals: issues and prospects. Brookings Institution. '67.

tamp, L. D. The geography of life and death. Cornell University Press. '65.

tamp, L. D. Some aspects of medical geography. Oxford University Press. '64.

'unley, Roul. The American health scandal. Harper. '66.

United States. Task Force on Medicaid and Related Programs. Report. Supt. of Docs. Washington, D.C. 20402. '70.

Veisbrod, B. A. Economics of public health. University of Pennsylvania Press. '61.

Villiams, Greer. Virus hunters. Knopf. '59.

Vright, Helen and Rapport, S. B. eds. The amazing world of medicine. Harper. '61.

'ost, Edward. U.S. health industry: the costs of acceptable medical care by 1975. Praeger. '69.

PERIODICALS

America. 122:177. F. 21, '70. Inflated health insurance costs.

*America. 122:406-11. Ap. 18, '70. Reforming the abortion laws: a doctor looks at the case. Denis Cavanagh.

America. 122:490-1. My. 9, '70. Open letter to American doctors: the abortion responsibility.

America. 123:56-7. Ag. 8, '70. Right to live. J. R. Quinn.

America. 123:168. S. 19, '70. Crisis of health care.

American Scholar. 39:694+. Autumn '70. Failure of American medicine. M. G. Michaelson.

Better Homes and Gardens. 48:48-9. N. '70. Is there any way out of our health care mess? Fred Bailey.

*Bulletin of the Atomic Scientists. 26:21-2. Ja. '70. Social consequences of new developments in medicine. Alexander Leaf.

*Business Week. p 50-1+. Ja. 17, '70. $60-billion crisis over medical care.

Business Week. p 26-7. Ap. 4, '70. Medical inflation goes under the knife.

Business Week. p 27. Je. 6, '70. Medicare kills off its cost predictor.

Business Week. p 82+. Jl. 25, '70. Grim diagnosis for medical schools.

Business Week. p 119. S. 12, '70. Executive health: the dangers of a stroke.

*Carnegie Quarterly. 18:1-12. Summer '70. Extreme remedies a: very appropriate for extreme diseases; American health care i: crisis.

Catholic World. 212:74-7. N. '70. Perverse observations on abo: tion. P. J. Weber.

Changing Times. 24:27-30. F. '70. Caution! These products ca: kill!

Changing Times. 24:15-18. Je. '70. Time to check over your healt insurance.

Christian Century. 87:228-9. F. 25, '70. Inflation and ideolog: physicians' abuse of Medicaid systems.

Christian Century. 87:624-31. My. 20, '70. Is abortion a righ: symposium.

Christian Century. 87:756-8. Je. 17, '70. Violence and nonviolenc in the cure of disease and the healing of patients. Michae Wilson.

Christian Century. 87:883. Jl. 22, '70. Medical justice [editorial].

Christianity Today. 14:24-5. Je. 5, '70. War on the womb.

Commentary. 49:59-66. Je. '70. In sickness and in health. E. J Cassell.

Commonweal. 92:131-2. Ap. 24, '70. Abortion debate.

Commonweal. 92:154. My. 1, '70. Anti-abortion lobby. John Deed:

Commonweal. 92:243-5. D. 4, '70. Health crisis. E. T. Chase.

Dun's Review. 95:51-2+. Ap. '70. Can companies reduce heart a: tacks? Janet Smith.

Ebony. 25:42-6+. Ap. '70. New spirit at old Meharry: cooperatio: with Taborian hospital in Mound Bayou, Miss.

Ebony. 25:81-4+. Je. '70. Flying black medics.

*Editorial Research Reports. 2, no 3:529-42. Jl. 15. '70. Stress i: modern life. William Gerber.

Editorial Research Reports. 2, no 4:545-62. Jl. 24, '70. Abortior law reform. R. L. Worsnop.

Electronics World. 83:25-7. F. '70. Electronics and the heart. F. W Holder.

Esquire. 73:118-19+. Ap. '70. I can afford to be sick. W. A. Nolen

Farm Journal. 93:24-5+. O. '69. Do animal fats cause heart attacks: D. Braun.

Forbes. 106:42. O. 1, '70. That queasy feeling: health insuranc: companies and government-supported health insurance.

orbes. 106:76+. O. 15, '70. Making hospitals pay; chain-operated-for-profit hospitals.

Fortune. 81:80-3+. Ja. '70. Better care at less cost without miracles. E. K. Faltermayer.

Fortune. 81:84-9+. Ja. '70. Change begins in the doctor's office. Dan Cordtz.

Fortune. 81:96-9+. Ja. '70. Hospitals need management even more than money. J. M. Mecklin.

Good Housekeeping. 170:64-5+. Ja. '70. Controversy over the pill. Bill Surface.

Good Housekeeping. 170:68-71+. F. '70. Why you really can't get good medical care. Charles Remsberg and Bonnie Remsberg.

Good Housekeeping. 171:59+. Jl. '70. What to do if the doctor comes. J. K. Lubold.

Good Housekeeping. 171:181. O '70. Copper bracelets for arthritis: fraud or cure?

Harper's Magazine. 240:92-9. Ap. '70. Right not to be born. M. K. Sanders.

Harvard Business Review. 48:65-74. S. '70. New blood for tired hospitals. R. G. Wasyluka.

Life. 68:38-48. Ja. 23, '70. Soviet medicine: report on the surgeon-general, A. A. Vishnevsky, by Rudolph Chelminski. Bill Ray.

Life. 68:20B-9. F. 27, '70. Abortion comes out of the shadows; with an anonymous interview, ed. by F. von Moschzisker.

Life. 68:22. F. 27, '70. The doctor was short, pleasant, and in a big hurry.

*Life. 68:48-50+. My. 29, '70. Dilemma in Dyersville—help wanted: doctors needed in a real nice Iowa town with a brand-new hospital, fine schools and a future. Loudon Wainwright.

Life. 68:67-8+. Je. 12, '70. Once a medic, now a medex.

Life. 69:68-72. O. 2, '70. Parting shots: what doctors think of their patients.

Life. 69:60-2+. O. 23, '70. Child called Noah. Josh Greenfeld.

Life. 69:24-31. N. 6, '70. Shock room: traumatic shock treatment at Houston's Ben Taub general.

Mental Hygiene. 54:155-8. Ja. '70. Perspective on community mental health and community psychiatry. F. H. Frankel.

Mental Hygiene. 54:172-9. Ja. '70. Community mental health: a new search for social orientation. J. S. Bockoven.

Mental Hygiene. 54:221-9. Ap. '70. Mental hospital patient-con sumer as a determinant of services. Toaru Ishiyama.

Mental Hygiene. 54:230-40. Ap. '70. Struggle for patients' rights i a state hospital. L. C. Suchotliff and others.

Mental Hygiene. 54:316-20. Ap. '70. Community in community mental health. E. B. Back.

Mental Hygiene. 54:337-46. Jl. '70. Case studies of volunteer pro grams in mental health. L. J. Cowne.

Mental Hygiene. 54:357-63. Jl. '70. Education of the community mental health assistant: dovetailing theory with practice. M E. Danzig.

Mental Hygiene. 54:364-9. Jl. '70. Mental health professionals' hang-ups in training mental health counselors. D. S. Shapiro.

Mental Hygiene. 54:370-3. Jl. '70. Patients helping patients; friend ship club at Boulder mental health center. Donna Hawxhurst and Hank Walzer.

Mental Hygiene. 54:447-9. Jl. '70. Effects of the Baltimore riots on psychiatric hospital admissions. G. D. Klee and Kurt Gorwitz.

Mental Hygiene. 54:498-502. O. '70. Hospitalizing the young: is it for their own good? H. H. Weiss and E. F. Pizer.

Nation. 210:69-70. Ja. 26, '70. Number one method.

Nation. 210:557-60. My. 11, '70. Commercializing the aged. R. E. Burger.

Nation. 210:680-3. Je. 8, '70. Insurance is not enough. G. A. Silver.

*National Observer. p 1+. N. 16, '70. Sick medical schools receive emergency help. Jim Hampton.

National Review. 22:1366-7. D. 15, '70. Catholics and abortion. W. F. Buckley, Jr.

Natural History. 79:60-7. N. '70. Healing in the Sierra Madre. David Werner.

*New Republic. 162:15-18. Ja. 17; 13-16. Ja. 24; 17-19. F. 7, '70. The growing pains of medical care. Fred Anderson.
        Discussion. New Republic. 162:36-9. Mr. 21, '70.

New Republic. 162:10-11. My. 2, '70. Will Finch flinch? prepay ment plan.

New Republic. 163:15-17. Jl. 11, '70. Alive but not well. Mal Schecter.

New Republic. 164:8. F. 27, '71. Here we come, Otto.

New York Times. p 33. Je. 7, '70. Health unit plan gains in Senate. R. D. Lyons.

New York Times. p 41. O. 16, '70. The miseducation of doctors. Michael Crichton.

New York Times. p 1+. O. 30, '70. Medical schools urged to train more doctors and alter fundamental goals.

New York Times. p 16. O. 30, '70. Excerpts from the Carnegie Commission's report on medical education in U.S.

New York Times. p 16. O. 30, '70. Flexner's attack closed "quack" schools quickly.

New York Times. p 24, Ja. 4, '71. Nixon plans to propose overhaul of health services that would seek to involve the private sector.

New York Times. p 1+. Ja. 6, '71. Law lets U.S. pay physicians who enlist to serve in slums. R. D. Lyons.

New York Times. p 29. Ja. 21, '71. Deaths in Chicago tied to poor care. Nancy Hicks.

New York Times. p 11. Ja. 30, '71. Medicare-Medicaid funds rise, but new programs seem vague. R. D. Lyons.

New York Times. p 1+. F. 3, '71. President to ask Medicare fee rise and benefit cuts. R. D. Lyons.

New York Times. p 1+. F. 19, '71. Nixon's health care plan proposes employers pay $2.5-billion more a year. R. D. Lyons.

New York Times. p 16. F. 19, '71. Excerpts from the President's message urging "a new national health strategy." R. M. Nixon.

New York Times. p 36. F. 19, '71. Mr. Nixon's health plan; editorial.

New York Times. p 34. Mr. 14, '71. National health insurance is expected in 3 years. R. D. Lyons.

New York Times. p 36. Mr. 14, '71. Growing use of mind-affecting drugs stirs concern. L. K. Altman.

New York Times. p 1+. Mr. 16, '71. Mills reported preparing U.S. health insurance bill. R. D. Lyons.

New York Times. p 1+. Mr. 28, '71. Ethics debate set off by life science gains. J. E. Brody and E. B. Fiske.

*New York Times. p 39. Ap. 2, '71. Myth and reality: problems of health care. E. L. Richardson.

New York Times. p 1+. Ap. 4, '71. Broader Medicare urged by U.S. Advisory Council. Marjorie Hunter.

New York Times. p 1+. Ap. 16, '71. Rockefeller asks a nonprofit setup for health care. Richard Severo.

New York Times. p 30. Ap. 16, '71. Aid plan in peril, physicians warn. H. M. Schmeck, Jr.

New York Times. p 34. Ap. 20, '71. Poor in Appalachia charge lack of medical care. R. D. Lyons.

New York Times. p 23. Ap. 26, '71. Guided missile techniques applied to artificial vision by coast scientists. E. R. Holles.

New York Times. p 26. Ap. 27, '71. Doctors find leukemia yielding to drug and radiation therapy. J. E. Brody.

New York Times. p 28. Ap. 27. '71. Health cost rise of 50% expected. R. D. Lyons.

New York Times. p 31. Ap. 28, '71. Nixon's health care proposal is altered and offered in House. R. D. Lyons.

New York Times. p 27. My. 3, '71. Medical teachers oppose separate U.S. cancer unit. H. M. Schmeck, Jr.

New York Times. p E 5. My. 9, '71. Death: making it easier for patient and family. J. E. Brody.

New York Times. p E 9. My. 9, '71. Medical school: a plan to get M.D.'s into the ghetto. F. M. Hechinger.

New York Times. p 1+. My. 12, '71. President vows to lead a drive against cancer. H. M. Schmeck, Jr.

New York Times. p 1+. Je. 11, '71. Backers of cancer agency nearing accord in Senate. H. M. Schmeck, Jr.

New York Times Magazine. p 30-1+. Ja. 25. '70. Constitutional question: is there a right to abortion? L. J. Greenhouse.

New York Times Magazine. p 7+. Je. 28, '70. After July 1, an abortion should be as simple to have as a tonsillectomy, but— L. J. Greenhouse.

New York Times Magazine. p 30-1+. O. 11, '70. Free clinic for street people; medical care without a hassle. Joseph Brenner.

Newsweek. 75:46. Mr. 9, '70. Abortion unlimited.

Newsweek. 75:65. Mr. 30, '70. Why VD is rising.

Newsweek. 75:53-6+. Ap. 13, '70. Abortion and the changing law.

Newsweek. 75:54-5. Ap. 13, '70. Whole world off her back; the Dorene Falk case.

Newsweek. 76:31. Jl. 13, '70. Matter of survival; hospital-construction bill.

Newsweek. 76:60. Jl. 13, '70. Abortions on demand.

Newsweek. 76:103. S. 14, '70. Hearts and palms.

Newsweek. 76:70. N. 9, '70. Calling Dr. Reform; proposals of the Carnegie Commission on Higher Education.

Newsweek. 76:62. N. 30, '70. How recession can kill.

ewsweek. 76:38-9. D. 28, '70. Fats and the heart; recommendations of the Inter-Society Commission for Heart Disease Resources.

Newsweek. 77:84-6+. F. 22, '71. The war on cancer: progress report.

arents Magazine. 45:35-7+. Ja. '70. What's ahead in medicine? M. R. Swift.

arents Magazine. 45:40-1+. Ag. '70. Family doctor: medicine's newest specialty. E. J. Kowalewski.

arents Magazine. 45:56-7. N. '70. Medical self-help: training for an emergency.

arents Magazine. 45:78-9. N. '70. How to get health insurance that's right for your family. Jack Galub.

TA Magazine. 64:19-20. My. '70. Heart in health and disease. L. W. Sauer.

amparts Magazine. 9:19-21. Ag. '70. Abortion reform: the new tokenism.

amparts Magazine. 9:26-31. N. '70. Kaiser: you pay your money and you take your chances. J. M. Carnoy.

eader's Digest. 96:155-8. Ja. '70. Beware those holiday accidents. J. H. Winchester.

Reader's Digest. 97:103-7. Jl. '70. Rx for the family-doctor shortage. W. C. Bornemeier.

edbook. 134:78-9+. Ap. '70. Abortion: a startling proposal. M. J. Halberstam.

edbook. 135:26+. My. '70. Report on venereal disease; ed. by Evelyn Jacobs. R. E. Rogers.

Saturday Review. 53:18-20. Ag. 22, '70. The "healthiest nation" myth. Abraham Ribicoff.

Saturday Review. 53:21-3+. Ag. 22, '70. Where doctors fail. J. H. Knowles.

aturday Review. 53:24-6+. Ag. 22, '70. Solving the doctor shortage. C. M. Cobb.

Saturday Review. 53:27-9+. Ag. 22, '70. Case for national health insurance. Rashi Fein.

aturday Review. 53:30-2. Ag. 22, '70. Can doctors cause disease? Norman Cousins.

aturday Review. 53:16-19+. S. 12, '70. Larry: case history of a mistake. R. M. McQueen.

aturday Review. 53:56-7. D. 19, '70. Our ailing medical schools. Leonard Baker.

Science. 169:267-8. Jl. 17, '70. Medical schools: portents of nation health insurance. John Walsh.

Science. 169:956-60. S. 4, '70. Health care: fund shortage imped training of medical aides. Joel Kramer.

Science. 170:713-14. N. 13, '70. Medical education: Carnegie par urges expansion acceleration. John Walsh.

Science Digest. 68:35-6. Jl. '70. Storefront psychiatry.

Science Digest. 68:61-4. Jl. '70. Your emotions: can they influen disease? H. B. Miller.

Science Digest. 68:75. S. '70. Seventeen-year-old invents heart-lu machine. S. V. Jones.

Science Digest. 68:75. N. '70. How's your paranoia?

Science News. 97:170. F. 14, '70. High cost of health.

Science News. 97:267-8. Mr. 14, '70. Revamping health care: pla ning ambulatory service.

*Science News. 97:276-7. Mr. 14, '70. Health care goes into t streets. Jeanne Bockel.

Science News. 97:430. My. 2, '70. Band-Aids and major surger

Science News. 97:480. My. 16, '70. Senate health care report.

Science News. 98:56. Jl. 25, '70. In epidemic proportions.

Science News. 98:363-4. N. 7, '70. Blueprint for reform of medic education; Carnegie Commission report.

Science News. 98:459. D. 19, '70. Conquest of cancer; propos national cancer authority.

Science News. 98:461. D. 19, '70. Role of diet; report of Inte Society Commission for Heart Disease Resources.

Scientific American. 222:50+. Ja. '70. Abortion and the courts.

Scientific American. 222:60. Mr. '70. Surge in surgery.

Scientific American. 222:15-23. Ap. '70. Delivery of medical ca S. R. Garfield.

Scientific American. 223:60. O. '70. When two hearts beat as tw

Senior Scholastic. 95:11-12. N. 3, '69. Should experimentation c prisoners be stopped? pro and con discussion.

*Senior Scholastic. 96:7-8. My. 4, '70. Abortion tumult.

Seventeen. 29:132-3+. Je. '70. What teenage medicine can do f you. Alice Lake.

Sports Illustrated. 33:37-41. Ag. 3, '70. Curious case of the copp band. Gilbert Cant.

ime. 95:34. Mr. 9, '70. Abortion on request: Hawaii.

ime. 95:54. Mr. 30, '70. Crisis in health care.

ime. 95:60+. Ap. 27, '70. Privacy and the psychiatrist.

ime. 95:68+. Ap. 27, '70. Transplant survival: L. B. Russell, Jr.

ime. 95:60-1. My. 11, '70. Insurance for the nation's health.

ime. 96:46+. Jl. 20, '70. Seductive patients.

Time. 96:36. Jl. 27, '70. V.D.: a national emergency.

ime. 96:43-4. O. 5, '70. State of Soviet medicine. Jerrold Schecter.

ime. 96:68. O. 12, '70. Debate over national health insurance.

ime. 96:38+. N. 9, '70. Curing the doctor shortage; Carnegie
Commission plan.

ime. 96:38. N. 9, '70. Paramedics: new doctors' helpers.

ime. 96:23. D. 28, '70. Death at the hospital.

oday's Education. 59:50-1. F. '70. Teaching about venereal
diseases. E. P. Vincent.

oday's Health. 48:20-3+. Mr. '70. New abortion laws: how are
they working? Theodore Irwin.

oday's Health. 48:38-41+. Ap. '70. Woman doctor is missing in
action. J. C. Hefley.

oday's Health. 48:34-5+. My. '70. How teens get a head start on
health careers. Arthur Henley.

oday's Health. 48:50-3+. My. '70. Meet the family doctor for the
'70's. Mike Michaelson.

Today's Health. 48:32-5. Je. '70. New clues in the virus-cancer
mystery. C. R. Goodheart and Barbara Goodheart.

oday's Health. 48:26-9+. Jl. '70. NHI is nigh; national health insurance plans. Linda Witt.

oday's Health. 48:13. Ag. '70. Engineers apply skills to medical
devices.

oday's Health. 48:64-5. O. '70. Who's who in the hospital? Viola
Anderson.

oday's Health. 48:41-3+. N. '70. Say it with a stomachache. Sally
Olds.

*Today's Health. 49:20-3+. Mr. '71. The "headache hunters" meet
the anxious American. W. B. Furlong.

U.S. News & World Report. 68:70-2. F. 16, '70. Medicare in trouble.

U.S. News & World Report. 68:68-73. F. 23, '70. Country's no.
health problem: interview. R. O. Egeberg.

U.S. News & World Report. 68:63. Mr. 16, '70. Behind rising co
of health care.

U.S. News & World Report. 68:62. Ap. 13, '70. Cheaper Medicar

*U.S. News & World Report. 68:87-9. Je. 15, '70. Will electroni
solve the doctor shortage?

U.S. News & World Report. 69:20-1. Jl. 6, '70. Machines to help tl
doctor.

U.S. News & World Report. 69:20-1. Jl. 6, '70. More progre
against the killer diseases.

*U.S. News & World Report. 69:26-9. Ag. 10, '70. Prepaid medic
care for all.

U.S. News & World Report. 69:29. Ag. 10, '70. National health ca
abroad.

U.S. News & World Report. 69:84-5. S. 14, '70. Whatever happene
to heart transplants?

U.S. News & World Report. 69:38-9. N. 2, '70. Threat to docte
supply: medical colleges going broke.

U.S. News & World Report. 69:46. D. 14, '70. Fighting disease: th
latest advances.

*U.S. News & World Report. 69:29. D. 28, '70. Good life vs. you
heart.

UNESCO Courier. 23:16-24. Mr. '70. Benefits to medicine: bioastr
nautics. Gene Gregory.

UNESCO Courier. 23:27-9. My. '70. Hidden factors in the geogr
phy of cancer. Nedd Willard.

Vital Speeches of the Day. 36:402-7. Ap. 15, '70. On the life science
address, March 5, 1970. Jean Mayer.

Vital Speeches of the Day. 36:478-80. My. 15, '70. Health care cost
address, April 8, 1970. J. J. Powers, Jr.

Vital Speeches of the Day. 36:549-53. Jl. 1, '70. Crime of abortion
address, April 9, 1970. B. F. Brown.

Vital Speeches of the Day. 36:632-4. Ag. 1, '70. Revolution i
medical care; address, June 24, 1970. W. C. Bornemeier.

Vital Speeches of the Day. 37:14-16. O. 15, '70. National healt
insurance; labor's no. 1 legislative goal; address, Sept. 7, 197(
George Meany.

Vital Speeches of the Day. 37:100-2. D. 1, '70. The health security program; medicine in the free enterprise system; address, Sept. 9, 1970. Paul Ashton.

'ogue. 156:144-5. N. 15, '70. What is a nervous breakdown? Elizabeth Kendall and Allene Talmey.

Wall Street Journal. p 1. Ja. 6, '71. Our daily bread. Mary Bralove.

Wall Street Journal. p 1+. Ja. 8, '71. Malpractice suits rise, lead doctors to treat patients with caution. Ellen Graham.